Pathophysiology

for B Pharmacy Students

As per the latest syllabus prescribed by Pharmacy Council of India

Course code: BP 204T Pathophysiology-Theory (Semester II)

Pathophysiology
for B Pharmacy Students

As per the latest syllabus prescribed by Pharmacy Council of India

Course code: BP 204T Pathophysiology-Theory (Semester II)

Ramesh Kumar Marya

MBBS, MD (Physiology), PhD (Physiology)

former
Professor and Head
Department of Physiology
AIMST University, Malaysia

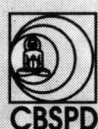

CBSPD

CBS Publishers & Distributors Pvt Ltd

New Delhi • Bengaluru • Chennai • Kochi • Kolkata • Lucknow • Mumbai
Hyderabad • Jharkhand • Nagpur • Patna • Pune • Uttarakhand

Pathophysiology
for B Pharmacy Students

ISBN: 978-93-90046-01-0

First Edition: 2020
Reprint 2022, 2024 2026.

Published by Satish Kumar Jain and produced by Varun Jain for
CBS Publishers & Distributors Pvt Ltd
4819/XI Prahlad Street, 24 Ansari Road, Daryaganj, New Delhi 110 002, India
Ph: 011-23289259, 23266861, 23266867   Fax: 011-23243014
Website: www.cbspd.com   e-mail: delhi@cbspd.com; cbspubs@airtelmail.in

Corporate Office: 204 FIE, Industrial Area, Patparganj, Delhi 110 092, India
Ph: 011-49344934   Fax: 011-49344935   e-mail: publishing@cbspd.com; publicity@cbspd.com

Branches

- **Bengaluru:** Seema House 2975, 17th Cross, K.R. Road, Banasankari 2nd Stage, Bengaluru 560 070, Karnataka, India
  Ph: +91-80-26771678/79   Fax: +91-80-26771680   e-mail: bangalore@cbspd.com
- **Chennai:** 7, Subbaraya Street, Shenoy Nagar, Chennai 600 030, Tamil Nadu, India
  Ph: +91-44-26680620, 26681266   Fax: +91-44-42032115   e-mail: chennai@cbspd.com
- **Kochi:** 42/1325, 1326, Power House Road, Opposite KSEB, Power House, Ernakulum 682018, Kochi, Kerala, India
  Ph: +91-484-4059061-67   Fax: +91-484-4059065   e-mail: kochi@cbspd.com
- **Kolkata:** 147, Hind Ceramics Compound, 1st Floor, Nilgunj Road, Belghoria, Kolkata 700056, West Bengal, India
  Ph: +91-33-25330055/56   e-mail: kolkata@cbspd.com
- **Lucknow:** Basement, Khushuma Complex, 7 Meerabai Marg (behind Jawahar Bhawan), Lucknow 226001, UP, India
  Ph: +91-522-40000032   e-mail: tiwari.lucknow@cbspd.com
- **Mumbai:** PWD Shed, Gala No. 25/26, Ramchandra Bhatt Marg, Next JJ Hospital Gate No. 2, Opp. Union Bank of India, Noorbaug, Mumbai 400009, Maharashtra, India
  Ph: +91-22-66661880/89   e-mail: mumbai@cbspd.com

Representatives

• **Hyderabad**	0-9885175004	• **Jharkhand**	0-9811541605	• **Nagpur**	0-9421945513
• **Patna**	0-9334159340	• **Pune**	0-9623451994	• **Uttarakhand**	0-9716462459

Printed at: Mudrak, Noida, UP, India.

Preface

The discipline of pharmacy is the science of preparing, dispensing, and reviewing drugs. It is a health profession that links health sciences with pharmaceutical sciences and aims to ensure the safe, and effective use of drugs. While dispensing drugs to the patients safely, rationally and effectively, a pharmacist needs to be fully aware of disorder for which a drug is being dispensed. It means that a pharmacist has to be familiar with aetiology, signs and symptoms, pathogenesis and complications of the disorder. A knowledge of pathogenesis and pathophysiology of a disorder not only helps in clear understanding of the mechanism of disease and its complications, but also creates a base for the rationale of the pharmacologic treatment.

This book has been written strictly according to the syllabus laid down recently by the Pharmacy Council of India for the course in pathophysiology in Semester II of Bachelor of Pharmacy course. The book has been written in a concise and student-friendly style. The description of various diseases has been written in such a simple language that a student of B Pharmacy course would not be deterred by high-sounding medical jargon. A large number of simple illustrations shall help in making the text clear.

I am thankful to CBS Publishers & Distributors for their keen interest in the publication of this book. Special thanks are due to Mr YN Arjuna, Senior Vice-President (Publishing, Editorial & Publicity), and his team for the beautiful layout of the text and illustrations. I invite suggestions from the teachers as well as the students for further improvement of the book.

Ramesh Kumar Marya

Contents

BP 204T Pathophysiology (Theory)

45 Hours

Scope: Pathophysiology is the study of causes of diseases and reactions of the body to such disease producing causes. This course is designed to impart a thorough knowledge of the relevant aspects of pathology of various conditions with reference to its pharmacological applications, and understanding of basic pathophysiological mechanisms. Hence, it will not only help to study the syllabus of pathology, but also to get baseline knowledge required to practice medicine safely, confidently, rationally and effectively.

Objectives: Upon completion of the subject student shall be able to:
1. Describe the etiology and pathogenesis of the selected disease states;
2. Name the signs and symptoms of the diseases; and
3. Mention the complications of the diseases.

< **COURSE CONTENT** >

Unit I	10 Hours

- **Basic principles of cell injury and adaptation:** Introduction, definitions, homeostasis, components and types of feedback systems, causes of cellular injury, pathogenesis (cell membrane damage, mitochondrial damage, ribosome damage, nuclear damage), morphology of cell injury—adaptive changes (atrophy, hypertrophy, hyperplasia, metaplasia, dysplasia), cell swelling, intra-cellular accumulation, calcification, enzyme leakage and cell death acidosis & alkalosis, electrolyte imbalance
- **Basic mechanism involved in the process of inflammation and repair:** Introduction, clinical signs of inflammation, different types of inflammation, mechanism of inflammation—alteration in vascular permeability and blood flow, migration of WBCs, mediators of inflammation, basic principles of wound healing in the skin, pathophysiology of atherosclerosis

Unit II	10 Hours

- **Cardiovascular system:** Hypertension, congestive heart failure, ischemic heart disease (angina, myocardial infarction, atherosclerosis and arteriosclerosis)
- **Respiratory system:** Asthma, chronic obstructive airways diseases.
- **Renal system:** Acute and chronic renal failure.

Unit III   10 Hours

- **Haematological diseases:** Iron deficiency, megaloblastic anemia (Vit B12 and folic acid), sickle cell anemia, thalassemia, hereditary acquired anemia, hemophilia
- **Endocrine system:** Diabetes, thyroid diseases, disorders of sex hormones
- **Nervous system:** Epilepsy, Parkinson's disease, stroke, psychiatric disorders: Depression, schizophrenia and Alzheimer's disease.
- **Gastrointestinal system:** Peptic ulcer

Unit IV   8 Hours

- **Inflammatory bowel diseases, jaundice, hepatitis (A, B, C, D, E, F), alcoholic liver disease.**
- **Disease of bones and joints:** Rheumatoid arthritis, osteoporosis and gout
- **Principles of cancer:** Classification, etiology and pathogenesis of cancer
- **Diseases of bones and joints:** Rheumatoid arthritis, osteoporosis, gout
- **Principles of cancer:** Classification, etiology and pathogenesis of cancer

Unit V   7 Hours

- **Infectious diseases:** Meningitis, typhoid, leprosy, tuberculosis
- **Urinary tract infections**
- **Sexually transmitted diseases:** AIDS, syphilis, gonorrhea

Basic Principles of Cell Injury and Adaptation

Definitions

➢ *Aetiology* is the origin of a disease, including the underlying causes and modifying factors.

➢ *Pathogenesis* refers to the steps in the development of disease. It describes how aetiologic factors trigger cellular and molecular changes that give rise to the specific functional and structural abnormalities of the disease. Whereas aetiology refers to *why* a disease arises, pathogenesis describes *how* a disease develops.

➢ **Pathology** describes the structural changes observed in a diseased tissue or an organ.

➢ **Pathophysiology** describes the biochemical, and functional changes that occur in cells, tissues, and organs in response to injury.

➢ **Morphology** describes changes in the gross (naked-eye) or microscopic appearance of a tissue or an organ.

Symptoms and Signs

A **symptom** is a subjective *feeling* of a departure from normal function which is apparent to *a patient*, reflecting the presence of an unusual state, or of a disease. A symptom can be subjective (felt by the patient) or objective (seen by the patient). Tiredness is a subjective symptom, whereas cough or fever are objective symptoms. In contrast to a symptom, a **sign** is a clue to a disease elicited *by an examiner or a doctor*. For example, edema feet is a sign of congestive heart failure or liver failure.

◁ HOMEOSTASIS ▷

The mammalian cells are very sensitive. The cells survival and function is dependent on the maintenance of the internal environment. The composition of internal environment may be disturbed by a variety of external or internal factors. Examples of external factors that may disturb internal environment include exposure to extremes of heat or cold, absence of food, deficiency of oxygen, etc. Examples of internal factors that may disturb internal environment include infections, blood loss, and increased utilization of glucose and production of excess of lactic acid by vigorously contracting muscles during severe exercise, etc. In all such conditions, various organs of the body maintain homeostasis, that is, act in a harmonious fashion and prevent marked changes in the physical and chemical composition of extracellular fluid. Failure of homeostatic mechanism results in disturbed body function known as disease.

HOMEOSTATIC MECHANISMS

As mentioned above, various physiological or pathological processes tend to disturb one or more components of internal environment. The disturbance sets into motion a series of physiological responses that eliminate the disturbing factor and normalize the composition of extracellular fluid (Fig. 1.1). The homeostatic mechanisms allow an organism to function effectively in a broad range of environmental conditions.

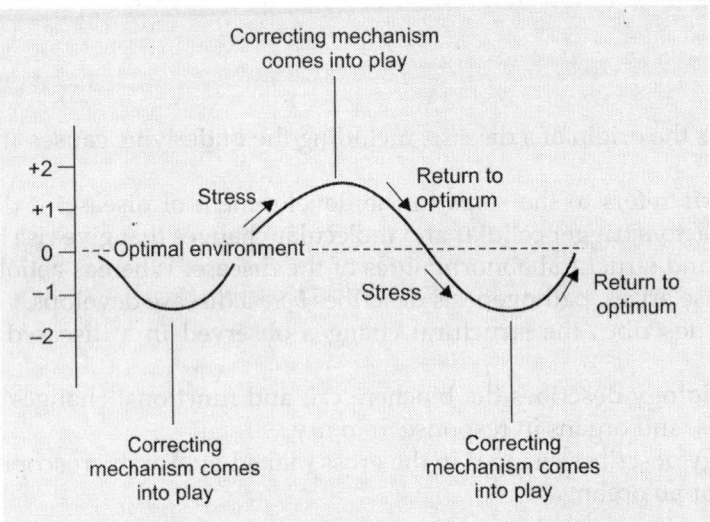

Fig. 1.1: Basic homeostatic mechanism of homeostasis

All homeostatic mechanisms have at least three components (Fig. 1.2):
1. **Receptor** that detects a change in the internal environment and sends information to the control center.
2. **Control center** is the structure that evaluates the disturbance and activates the correcting mechanisms.
3. **Effector** is the structure that carries out the corrective responses as directed by the control center.

For example, exposure to cold tends to lower the body temperature. The change in body temperature is detected by cold thermal receptors **(receptor)**. The information is communicated to the temperature-regulating areas of hypothalamus in the brain **(center)**. The body responds by involuntary contractions of skeletal muscle called shivering **(effector)**. Shivering generates heat and prevents a fall in body temperature. Exposure to hot environment tends to raise body temperature. The change in body temperature is detected by warmth thermal receptors **(receptor)**. The information is communicated to the temperature-regulating areas of hypothalamus in the brain **(center)**. The body responds by sweating that results in heat loss by evaporation **(effector)**. This is an example of **body temperature homeostasis**.

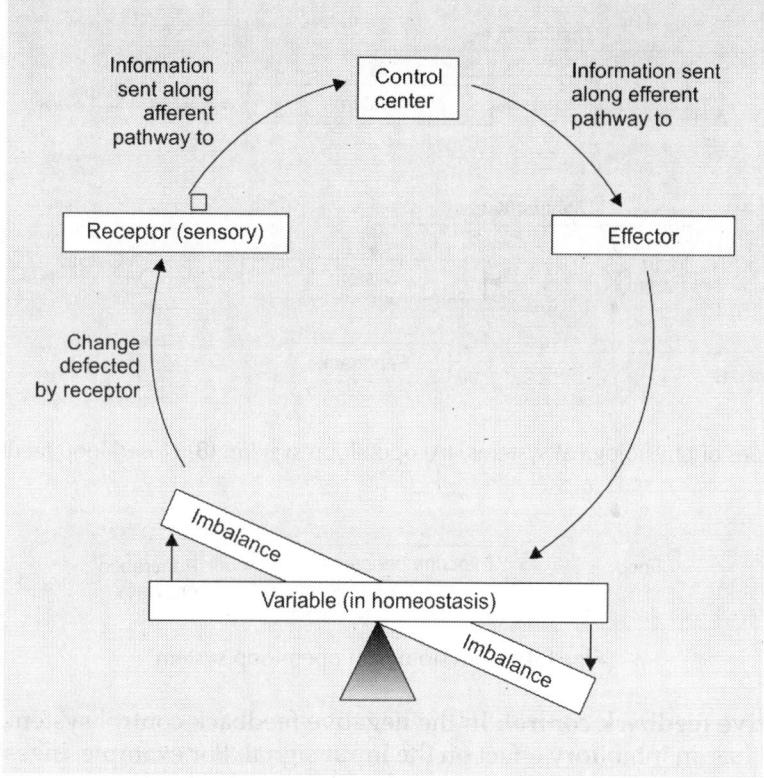

Fig. 1.2: Components of homeostatic mechanisms

PHYSIOLOGICAL CONTROL SYSTEMS

Our body consists of many *organ systems,* and each organ system consists of more than one organ. Therefore, central control mechanisms are required so as to allow coordination of activity of different organs of an organ system and coordination between different organ systems. Our body has two major control systems.

   A. **Neural control:** It is chiefly exerted on skeletal muscles and exocrine glands. The response occurs in milliseconds.
   B. **Endocrine control:** It is chiefly exerted on metabolic reactions. The response may take seconds, hours or even days.

   Open-loop and closed-loop processes (systems). Physiological processes may be governed by an open-loop system or a closed-loop system. In an open-loop system, the output product (signal) has no control over the process. The entire process is controlled by the input signals (Fig. 1.3A). In a closed-loop control, the product in the system (output signal) has an effect on the input signal (Fig. 1.3B). This is called a feedback phenomenon. Feedback control may be a negative feedback or a positive feedback system.

   1. **Open-loop system:** Presence of food in the intestine results in secretion of enzymes from the pancreas. However, the concentration of pancreatic enzymes in the intestine has no effect on the secretion of pancreatic acini (Fig. 1.4). This is an example of open-loop system.

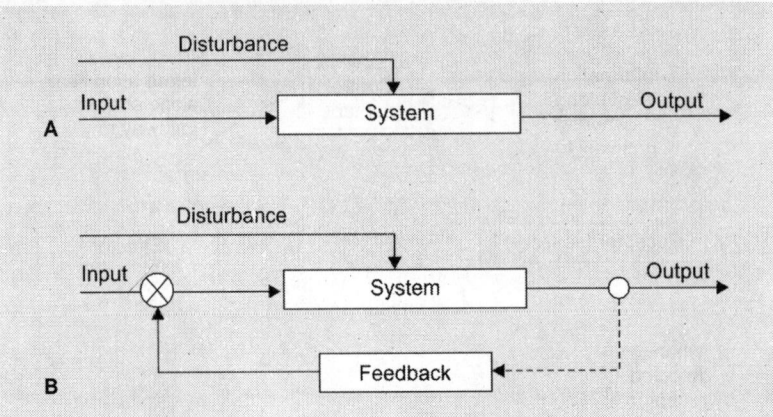

Fig. 1.3: Types of physiological systems. (A) open-loop system, (B) closed-loop feedback system

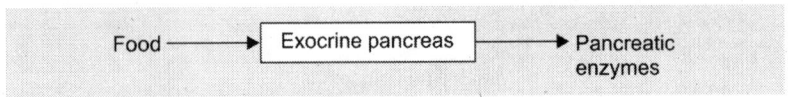

Fig. 1.4: A physiological open-loop system

2. **Negative feedback control:** In the negative feedback control system, the output signal has an inhibitory effect on the input signal. For example, ingestion of food results in secretion of gastric juice that contains hydrochloric acid (secreted by parietal cells of gastric glands). Secretion of acid has a negative feedback effect on parietal cells---- when the concentration of acid in gastric juice reaches a certain level (pH 2), the acidity has inhibitory effect on parietal cells and thus further acid secretion stops (Fig. 1.5). As a result, gastric acidity cannot increase beyond a certain predetermined degree. *Negative feedback control mechanisms are most often used in the maintenance of homeostasis.* This system prevents deviations from a given set point.

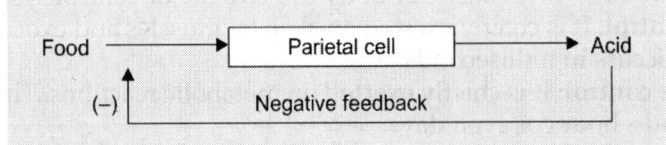

Fig. 1.5: A physiological closed-loop negative feedback system

3. **Positive feedback system:** In a positive feedback system, the output signal accentuates the input signal. As a result, the output deviates more and more from the initial output. Positive feedback system is not involved in homeostasis. It is used to accelerate or reinforce a reaction. For example, during delivery, at about 40 weeks of pregnancy, uterine contractions start that are weak to begin with. Mild uterine contractions cause pressure of head of the baby on the cervix and dilate it. Dilatation of the cervix reflexly causes release of a hormone oxytocin by the pituitary gland. Oxytocin causes stronger uterine contractions that cause

further dilatation of cervis and still greater release of oxytocin (Fig. 1.6). In this way, by a positive feedback mechanism, uterine contractions gradually become so strong that the baby is expelled out of the uterus.

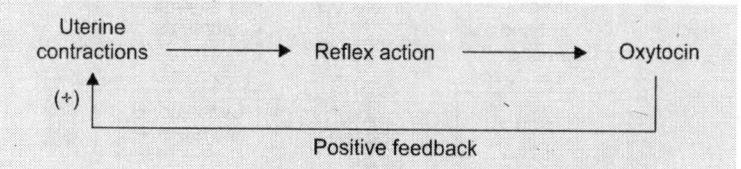

Fig. 1.6: A positive feedback system during delivery

4. **Feedforward system:** This system allows the human body to foresee a change in environment and prepares the body for the change. The information is sent ahead of time to the control system. The effector system is modified before any change has taken place, i.e. by anticipating change the environment (Fig. 1.7). Feedforward control system is advantageous in fast reactions. For example, during a cricket match, when a fielder tries to catch the ball, he has to anticipate the trajectory of the ball by visual input and run to an appropriate place. In most of the voluntary movements, both feedforward and negative feedback systems operate simultaneously.

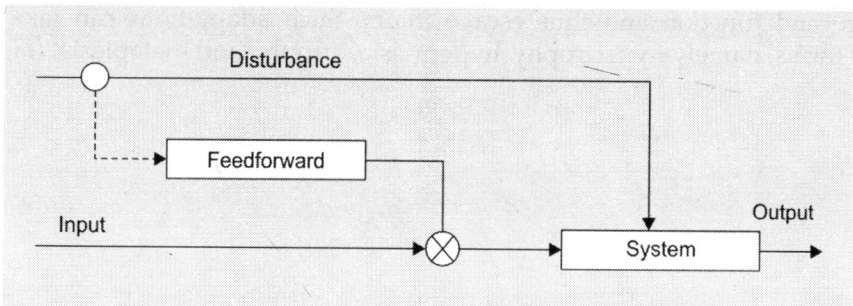

Fig. 1.7: Feedforward control system

CELLULAR RESPONSE TO PATHOLOGICAL STRESS OR NOXIOUS STIMULI

Cells or tissues encounter pathological stresses or stimuli, in the form of hypoxia, ischaemia, infections, and physical or chemical insults. The cells can respond to such stimuli by undergoing two fundamental processes:

1. **Adaptation,** modifying themselves to a new steady state and preserving viability and function. The principal adaptive responses are *hypertrophy, hyperplasia, atrophy,* and *metaplasia*.
2. **Cell injury:** If the stressful stimulus exceeds the adaptive capability, cell injury results. Depending on the strength of noxious stimulus, cell injury may be
   i. reversible and subsequently normal cellular function is restored, or
   ii. Irreversible, resulting in death of the cells or tissues (Fig. 1.8)

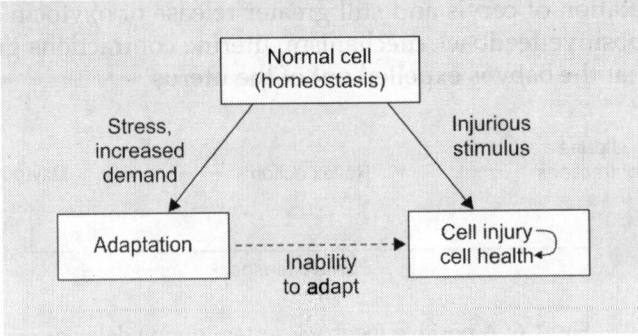

Fig. 1.8: Cellular responses to stressful or injurious stimuli

CELLULAR ADAPTATIONS TO STRESS

Adaptations are reversible changes in the number, size or metabolic activity of cells in response to changes in their environment.

Physiologic adaptations usually represent responses of cells to normal stimulation by hormones or endogenous chemical mediators (e.g. the hormone-induced enlargement of the breast and uterus during pregnancy).

Pathologic adaptations are responses to stress that allow cells to modulate their structure and function and thus escape injury. Such adaptations can take several distinct forms, namely hypertrophy, hyperplasia, atrophy and metaplasia. (Fig. 1.9)

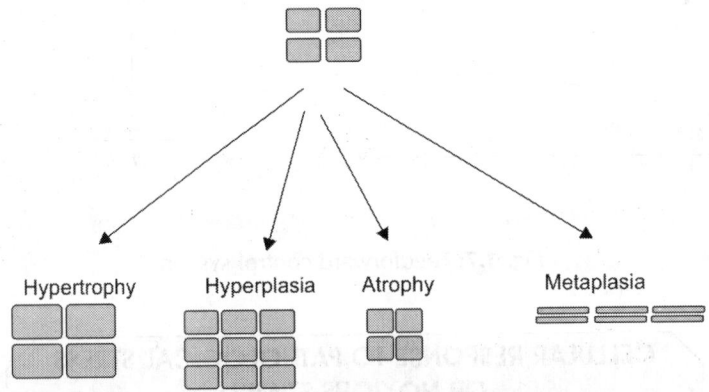

Fig. 1.9: Various types of pathologic adaptations in response to stress

▌HYPERTROPHY

Hypertrophy is an increase in the size of cells resulting in increase in the size of the organ. In pure hypertrophy there are no new cells, just bigger cells containing increased amounts of structural proteins and organelles. Hypertrophy occurs when cells have a limited capacity to divide. *Hypertrophy can be physiologic or pathologic* and is caused either by increased functional demand or by growth factor or hormonal stimulation. An example of physiologic hypertrophy is the enlarged muscle of the weightlifter. Thickening of ventricular muscle in response to narrowing of outlet valve is an example of pathologic hypertrophy (Fig. 1.10).

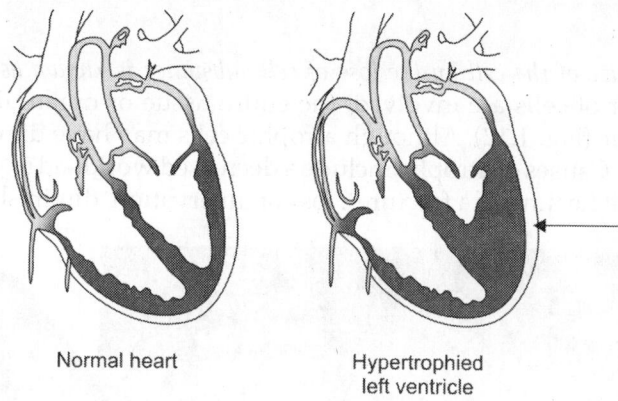

Normal heart   Hypertrophied
                                left ventricle

Fig. 1.10: Pathologic hypertrophy in the heart (arrow)

HYPERPLASIA

Hyperplasia is characterized by an increase in the size of an organ due to an *increase in cell number*. It results from a proliferation of tissue cells. Hyperplasia takes place if the tissue contains cell populations capable of replication; it may occur concurrently with hypertrophy and often in response to the same stimuli. *Hyperplasia can be physiologic or pathologic.*

An example of *physiologic hyperplasia* is the enlargement of mammary gland by proliferation of the glandular tissue during pregnancy and lactation (Fig.1.11). Benign prostatic hyperplasia leading to enlargement of prostate gland is an example of pathological hyperplasia.

An important point is that in all of these situations, *the hyperplastic process remains controlled; if the signals that initiate it disappear, the hyperplasia disappears.* It is this responsiveness to normal regulatory control mechanisms that distinguishes pathologic hyperplasia from cancer, in which the growth control mechanisms become dysregulated or ineffective.

Hypertrophy and hyperplasia can occur simultaneously. The massive physiologic enlargement of the uterus during pregnancy occurs as a consequence of oestrogen stimulated smooth muscle hypertrophy and smooth muscle hyperplasia.

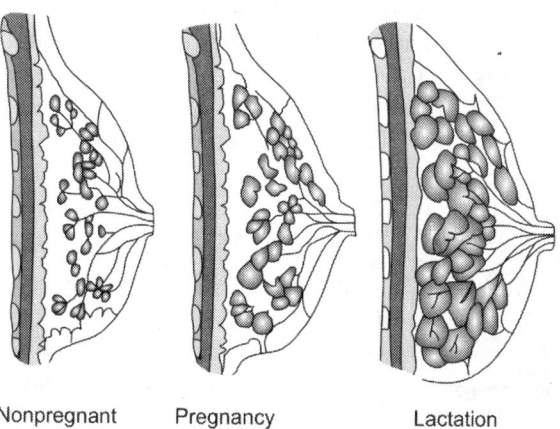

Nonpregnant   Pregnancy   Lactation

Fig. 1.11: Hyperplasia of mammary gland during pregnancy and lactation

ATROPHY

Shrinkage in the size of the cell by the loss of cell substance is known as atrophy. When a sufficient number of cells are involved, the entire tissue or organ diminishes in size, becoming atrophic (Fig. 1.12). Although atrophic cells may have diminished function, they are not dead. Causes of atrophy include a decreased workload (e.g. immobilization of a limb to permit healing of a fracture), loss of innervation, diminished blood supply,

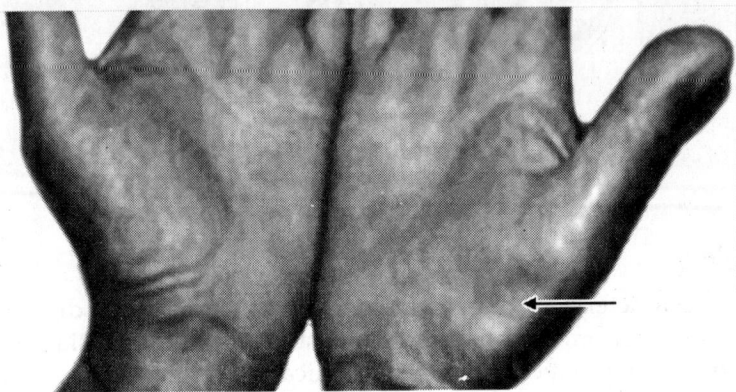

Fig. 1.12: Atrophy of the muscles of the palm of hand (arrow)

inadequate nutrition, loss of endocrine stimulation, and aging (senile atrophy). Although some of these stimuli are physiologic (e.g. the loss of hormone stimulation in menopause) and others pathologic (e.g. denervation). Cellular atrophy represents a retreat by the cell to a smaller size at which survival is still possible; a new equilibrium is achieved between cell size and diminished blood supply or nutrition.

METAPLASIA

Metaplasia is a reversible change in which one cell type (epithelial or mesenchymal) is replaced by another cell type. In this type of cellular adaptation, a cell type sensitive to a particular stress is replaced by another cell type that is better able to withstand the adverse environment. Epithelial metaplasia is exemplified by the change of normal stratified squamous epithelium of the lower end of oesophagus to intestinal columnar epithelium in patients of gastro-oesophageal reflux disease (GERD). In GERD, weak functioning of lower oesophageal sphincter leads to reflux of gastric acid into oesophagus. Chronic acid exposure converts stratified squamous epithelium to columnar epithelium (Fig. 1.13). Columnar epithelium is more resistant to acid.

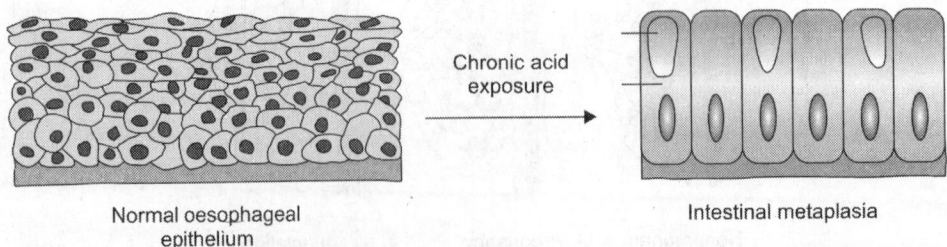

Normal oesophageal epithelium

Chronic acid exposure

Intestinal metaplasia

Fig. 1.13: Metaplasia in oesophageal epithelium

Another example is the metaplasia seen in the respiratory mucosa in chronic smokers. In this case the normal delicate ciliated columnar epithelial cells of the trachea and bronchi are focally replaced by more rugged stratified squamous epithelial cells. However, *the influences that induce metaplastic change, if persistent, may predispose to malignant transformation of the epithelium.*

CELL INJURY

Cell injury results when cells are stressed so severely that they are no longer able to adapt or when cells are exposed to inherently damaging agents or suffer from intrinsic abnormalities (e.g. in DNA or proteins). Different injurious stimuli affect many metabolic pathways and cellular organelles. Injury may progress through a reversible stage and culminate in irreversible change, i.e. cell death.

REVERSIBLE CELL INJURY

In early stages or mild forms of injury, the functional and morphologic changes are reversible if the damaging stimulus is removed. At this stage, although there may be significant structural and functional abnormalities, the injury has typically not progressed to severe membrane damage and nuclear dissolution.

IRREVERSIBLE CELL INJURY (CELL DEATH)

Cell death may occur in the form of (i) necrosis, or (ii) apoptosis

➤ **Necrosis:** With continuing damage, the injury becomes irreversible, at which time the cell cannot recover and it dies. When damage to membranes is severe, enzymes leak out of lysosomes, enter the cytoplasm, and digest the cell, resulting in *necrosis.* Cellular contents also leak through the damaged plasma membrane into the extracellular space, where they elicit a host reaction (inflammation). Necrosis is the major pathway of cell death in many commonly encountered injuries, such as those resulting from ischemia, exposure to toxins, various infections, and trauma.

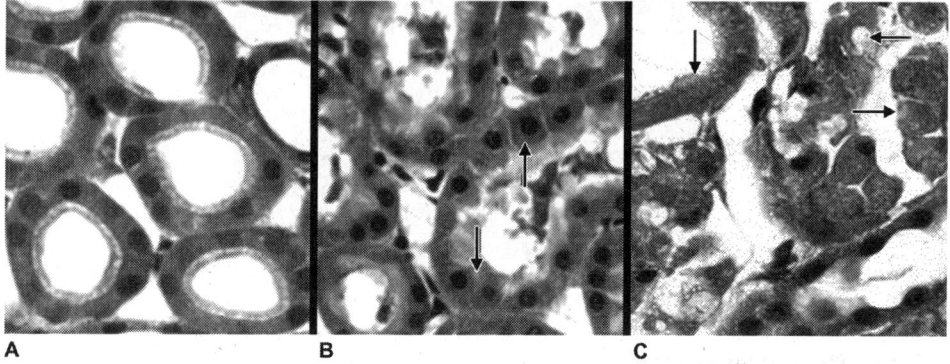

A   B   C

Fig. 1.14: Stages of response to cell injury. (A) Normal cells, (B) cellular swelling, (C) cellular necrosis

➤ **Apoptosis:** When a cell is deprived of growth factors, or the cell's DNA or proteins are damaged beyond repair, the cell kills itself by another type of death, called *apoptosis,* which is characterized by nuclear dissolution without complete loss of membrane integrity. *Whereas necrosis is always a pathologic process, apoptosis serves many normal functions and is not necessarily associated with pathologic cell injury. Furthermore, in keeping with its role in certain physiologic processes, apoptosis does not elicit an inflammatory response.* The morphologic features, mechanisms, and significance of these two death pathways are discussed in more detail later in this chapter.

Histologic Signs of Reversible Cell Injury

i. **Cellular swelling:** The first sign of almost all forms of injury to cells, is a reversible alteration called cellular swelling (Fig. 1.14B). Microscopic examination may reveal small, clear vacuoles within the cytoplasm; these represent distended and pinched-off segments of the endoplasmic reticulum (ER). This pattern of nonlethal injury is sometimes called **vacuolar degeneration.** The intracellular changes associated with reversible injury include:

   (1) plasma membrane alterations such as blunting, or distortion of microvilli, and loosening of intercellular attachments;

   (2) mitochondrial swelling

   (3) dilation of the ER with detachment of ribosomes and

   (4) minimal nuclear alterations (clumping of chromatin).

   Cellular swelling is the result of failure of energy-dependent ion pumps in the plasma membrane, leading to an inability to maintain ionic and fluid homeostasis.

ii. **Fatty change:** Fatty change occurs in hypoxic injury and in various forms of toxic or metabolic injury. It is manifested by the appearance of small or large lipid vacuoles in the cytoplasm (Fig. 1.15). It is principally encountered in cells participating in fat metabolism (e.g. hepatocytes). Like cellular swelling, fatty change is also reversible stage of tissue injury.

Normal liver   Fatty liver

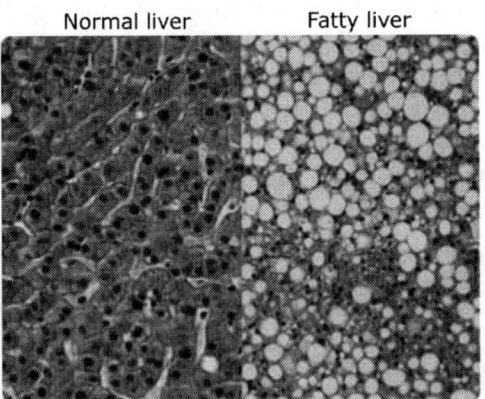

Fig. 1.15: Fatty change in the liver

Histologic Signs of Necrosis

Necrosis is the type of cell death that is associated with loss of membrane integrity and leakage of cellular contents culminating in dissolution of cells, largely resulting from the degradative action of enzymes on lethally injured cells (Fig. 1.14C). The leaked cellular contents often elicit a local host reaction, called *inflammation*, that attempts to eliminate the dead cells and start the subsequent repair process (Chapter 2). The enzymes responsible for digestion of the cell may be derived from the lysosomes of the dying cells themselves and from the lysosomes of leukocytes that are recruited as part of the inflammatory reaction to the dead cells

Necrosis is characterized by changes in the cytoplasm and nuclei of the injured cells

i. **Cytoplasmic changes**
   - ➤ Increased *eosinophilia* (deep pink staining in slides stained with H & E). It is attributable in part to increased binding of eosin to denatured cytoplasmic proteins and in part to loss of the basophilia that is normally imparted by the ribonucleic acid (RNA) in the cytoplasm.
   - ➤ Compared with viable cells, the cell may have a more *glassy, homogeneous* appearance, mostly because of the loss of glycogen particles.
   - ➤ When enzymes have digested cytoplasmic organelles, the cytoplasm becomes vacuolated and appears *"moth-eaten."*
   - ➤ By electron microscopy, necrotic cells are characterized by *discontinuities in plasma and organelle membranes,* marked *dilation of mitochondria* with the appearance of large amorphous densities and disruption of lysosomes.

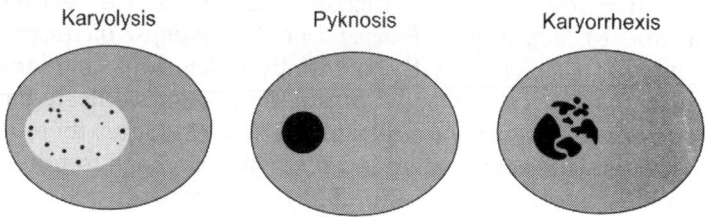

Fig. 1.16: Nuclear changes in necrosis

ii. **Nuclear changes:** Nuclear changes assume one of three patterns, all due to breakdown of DNA and chromatin (Fig. 1.16).
   - ➤ *Karyolysis,* in which basophilia of the chromatin may fade presumably secondary to deoxyribonuclease (DNase) activity.
   - ➤ *Pyknosis,* characterized by nuclear shrinkage and increased basophilia; the DNA condenses into a solid shrunken mass.
   - ➤ *Karyorrhexis,* the pyknotic nucleus undergoes fragmentation.

Fates of Necrotic Cells

- ➤ Necrotic cells may persist for some time or may be digested by enzymes and disappear.
- ➤ Dead cells may be phagocytosed by other cells
- ➤ Dead cells ultimately becoming **calcified**.

Mechanisms of Cell Injury

Cell injury results from functional and biochemical abnormalities in one or more of several essential cellular components. The principal targets and biochemical mechanisms of cell injury are:

1. Mitochondria and their ability to generate ATP and ROS under pathologic conditions
2. Disturbance in calcium homeostasis

3. Damage to cellular (plasma and lysosomal) membranes
4. Damage to DNA.

1. **ATP depletion:** The major causes of ATP depletion are reduced supply of oxygen and nutrients, as well as mitochondrial damage. ATP is required for virtually all synthetic and degradative processes within the cell, including membrane transport, protein synthesis, lipogenesis, etc. Deficiency of ATP leads to:
   a. Reduced activity of Na-K-ATPase pump resulting in intracellular accumulation of sodium and efflux of potassium. The net gain of solute is accompanied by gain of water, causing *cell swelling* and dilation of the endoplasmic reticulum.
   b. A compensatory *increase in anaerobic glycolysis* in an attempt to maintain the cell's energy sources. As a consequence, intracellular glycogen stores are rapidly depleted, and lactic acid accumulates, leading to decreased intracellular pH and decreased activity of many cellular enzymes.

2. **Influx of calcium:** Ischaemia and certain toxins cause an increase in cytosolic calcium concentration, initially because of release of Ca^{2+} from the intracellular stores, and later resulting from increased influx of Ca^{2+} across the plasma membrane due to *failure of ATP-dependent Ca^{2+} pumps. Increased cytosolic Ca^{2+} activates a number of enzymes,* with potentially deleterious cellular effects. There is *structural disruption of the protein synthetic apparatus,* manifested as detachment of ribosomes from the rough endoplasmic reticulum. Thus, there is reduction in protein synthesis. Ultimately, there is irreversible damage to mitochondrial and lysosomal membranes, and the cell undergoes necrosis.

3. **Defects in membrane permeability:** Increased membrane permeability leading ultimately to overt membrane damage is a consistent feature of most forms of cell injury that culminate in necrosis. The most important sites of membrane damage during cell injury are the mitochondrial membrane, the plasma membrane, and membranes of lysosomes.
   ➤ *Mitochondrial membrane damage.* Damage to mitochondrial membranes leads to further reduction in production of ATP culminating in necrosis.
   ➤ *Plasma membrane damage.* Plasma membrane damage leads to loss of osmotic balance and influx of fluids and ions, as well as loss of cellular contents.
   ➤ *Injury to lysosomal membranes* results in leakage of their enzymes into the cytoplasm and activation of the acid hydrolases in the acidic intracellular pH of the injured (e.g. ischaemic) cell. Lysosomes contain ribonucleases (RNAses), DNAses, proteases, glucosidases, and other enzymes. Activation of these enzymes leads to enzymatic digestion of cell components, and the cells die by necrosis.

4. **Damage to DNA:** Cells have mechanisms that repair damage to DNA, but if this damage is too severe to be corrected, the cell initiates its suicide program and dies by apoptosis.

◁ **APOPTOSIS** ▷

Apoptosis is a pathway of cell death in which cells activate enzymes that degrade the cells' own nuclear DNA and nuclear and cytoplasmic proteins. Fragments of the apoptotic cells then break off, giving the appearance that is responsible for the name (*apoptosis,* "falling off") (Fig. 1.17). The plasma membrane of the apoptotic cell remains intact, but the membrane is altered in such a way that the cell and its fragments become targets for phagocytes. The dead cell and its fragments are rapidly cleared before cellular contents have leaked out, so *apoptotic cell death does not elicit an inflammatory reaction in the host*. Apoptosis differs in this respect from necrosis, which is characterized by loss of membrane integrity, enzymatic digestion of cells, leakage of cellular contents, and frequently a host reaction. However, apoptosis and necrosis sometimes coexist, and apoptosis induced by some pathologic stimuli may progress to necrosis.

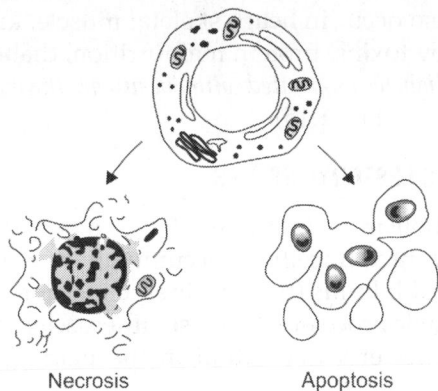

Necrosis   Apoptosis

Fig. 1.17: Necrosis and apoptosis

Causes of Apoptosis

Apoptosis occurs in many normal situations and serves to eliminate potentially harmful cells and cells that have outlived their usefulness. It also occurs as a pathologic event when cells are damaged beyond repair, especially when the damage affects the cell's DNA; in these situations, the irreparably damaged cell is eliminated by apoptosis.

Physiological Apoptosis

➢ *Involution of hormone-dependent tissues upon hormone deprivation*, such as endometrial cell breakdown during the menstrual cycle, and regression of the lactating breast after weaning.
➢ *Cell loss in proliferating cell populations*, such as intestinal crypt epithelia, in order to maintain a constant number.
➢ *Elimination of cells that have served their useful purpose*, such as neutrophils in an acute inflammatory response.

Pathologic Apoptosis

➢ *Damaged DNA*
➢ *Apoptosis eliminates cells that are genetically altered or injured beyond repair and does so without eliciting a severe host reaction, thereby keeping the extent of tissue damage to a minimum.* Death by apoptosis is responsible for loss of cells in a variety of pathologic states that damage the DNA of cells.
➢ *Cell injury in certain infections*, particularly viral infections, in which loss of infected cells is largely due to apoptotic death that may be induced by the virus.

<INTRACELLULAR ACCUMULATIONS>

Intracellular accumulations of various substances and extracellular deposition of calcium, both of which are often associated with cell injury.

FAT

Fatty change refers to any abnormal accumulation of triglycerides within parenchymal cells. It is most often seen in the liver, since this is the major organ involved in fat metabolism, but it may also occur in heart, skeletal muscle, kidney, and other organs. Steatosis may be caused by toxins, protein malnutrition, diabetes mellitus, obesity, or anoxia. *Alcohol abuse and diabetes associated with obesity are the most common causes of fatty change in the liver* (fatty liver) (Fig. 1.15).

CHOLESTEROL AND CHOLESTERYL ESTERS

Cellular cholesterol metabolism is tightly regulated to ensure normal cell membrane synthesis without significant intracellular accumulation. However, phagocytic cells may become overloaded with lipids (triglycerides, cholesterol, and cholesteryl esters) in several different pathologic processes. Of these, atherosclerosis is the most important. The role of lipid and cholesterol deposition in the pathogenesis of atherosclerotic plaque is discussed in Chapter 3.

GLYCOGEN

Excessive intracellular deposits of glycogen are associated with abnormalities in the metabolism of either glucose or glycogen. In poorly controlled diabetes mellitus, the prime example of abnormal glucose metabolism, glycogen accumulates in renal tubular epithelium, cardiac myocytes, and β cells of the islets of Langerhans (Fig. 1.18).

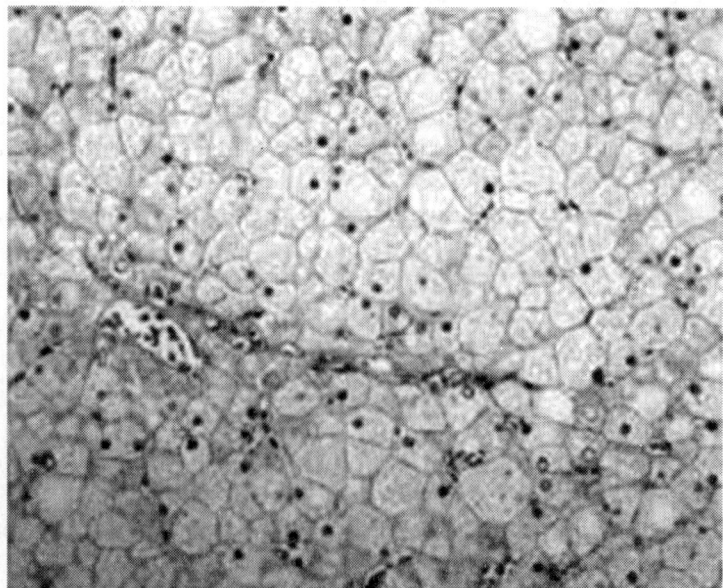

Fig. 1.18: Glycogen deposition in the hepatocytes in a case of diabetes mellitus

LIPOFUSCIN

It is an insoluble brownish-yellow granular intracellular material that accumulates in a variety of tissues (particularly the heart, liver, and brain) as a result of age or atrophy (Fig. 1.19).

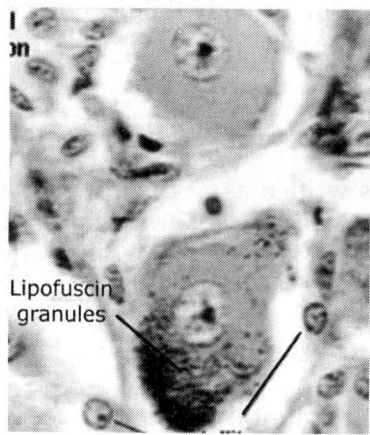

Lipofuscin granules

Fig. 1.19: Lipofuscin granules in a neuron

CALCIUM

Pathologic calcification is a common process in a wide variety of disease states; it implies the abnormal deposition of calcium salts. When the deposition occurs in dead or dying tissues, it is called *dystrophic calcification; it occurs in the absence of derangements in calcium metabolism,* i.e. with normal serum levels of calcium. In contrast, the deposition of calcium salts in normal tissues is known as *metastatic calcification and is almost always secondary to hypercalcaemia* (Fig. 1.20).

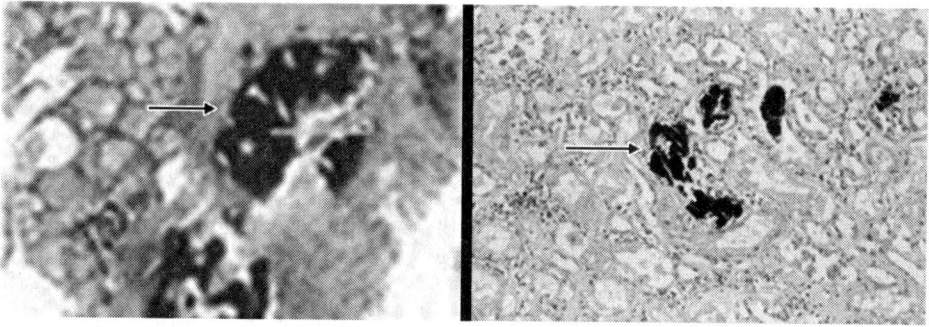

Fig. 1.20: Dystrophic (left) and metastatic calcification (right)

ACIDOSIS AND ALKALOSIS

THE CONCEPT OF pH

An **acid** is a chemical species that can donate a proton (H^+), and a **base** is a species that can accept (gain) a proton. Pure water undergoes extremely small degree of dissociation to yield H^+ and OH^-.

$$H_2O \leftrightarrow H^+ + OH^-$$

The concentration of H^+ in water is 10^{-7} mEq/L. Water is regarded as neutral. Acids are solutions with H^+ concentration greater than 10^{-7} (e.g. 10^{-6} or 10^{-5} mEq/L). Alkalis or bases are solutions with H^+ concentration less than 10^{-7} (e.g. 10^{-8} or 10^{-9} mEq/L). Expression of H^+ concentration in the body fluids as described above is cumbersome; hence a symbol pH came to be used:

$$pH = \log \frac{1}{\left[H^+\right]}$$

Thus pH of pure water is written as 7. The arterial blood has an average pH of 7.4 (normal range 7.35–7.45). A decrease of arterial pH value below 7.35 is known as acidosis, whereas the term alkalosis is used to describe arterial pH values higher than 7.45. Arterial pH value below 6.8 or above 8 is not compatible with life. In fact, arterial pH is maintained within a narrow range, transiently with the help of acid–base buffers in the body fluids, and finally by the kidneys and the lungs.

Regulation of Hydrogen Ion Balance

➤ Buffer systems response—very rapid (in seconds), incomplete
➤ Respiratory responses—rapid (in minutes), incomplete
➤ Renal responses—slow (in hours to days), complete

Under normal circumstances, tremendous amounts of hydrogen ions (H^+) are being continuously added to the body fluids. Carbon dioxide accounts for the addition of over 12,000 mEq H^+ per day. Nonvolatile (fixed) acids account for another 60 mEq/day. Almost all the CO_2 is excreted by the lungs, whereas the kidney is responsible for the excretion of non-volatile acid products of protein metabolism. Lactic acid produced during severe exercise or keto acids produced in severe diabetes are also excreted by the kidney.

Fruits are the main dietary source of the alkali. They contain sodium and potassium salts of weak organic acids, whose metabolism produces $NaHCO_3$ or $KHCO_3$ (and CO_2). Normally, the alkali content of the diet is very small and all the normal individuals excrete acidic urine except for transient post-prandial alkaline tide.

| ROLE OF RESPIRATION

In response to changes in blood pH, respiratory responses occur within minutes by stimulation/depression of respiratory centers in the CNS.

In spite of addition of 12,000 mEq H^+ per day to the blood, the pH of arterial blood remains remarkably constant at 7.4. Similarly pCO_2 of the arterial blood is kept constant at 40 mm Hg. This is made possible by two factors:

i. In the venous blood, CO_2 is converted to H_2CO_3 and further to H^+ and HCO_3^-. Hydrogen ions are immediately buffered by the blood buffers, chiefly haemoglobin and plasma proteins.

ii. As the venous blood passes through the lungs, CO_2 is regenerated by reversal of the reactions mentioned above (i) and excreted very efficiently. The pulmonary ventilation is so delicately adjusted that it exactly matches the CO_2 produced in the body. Even during severe exercise, when CO_2 production increases 20 folds, CO_2 excretion is so efficient that arterial pCO_2 does not increase at all. Such a delicate control is made possible by the fact that ventilation is controlled by both CO_2 as well as H^+ concentration through central and peripheral chemoreceptors.

 a. *Effect of CO_2:* CO_2 is a highly diffusible gas. It can easily cross the blood–brain and blood–CSF barriers, and stimulate the medullary central chemoreceptors. In contrast, H^+ cannot cross these barriers easily. Therefore, central chemoreceptors are most sensitive to changes in arterial pCO_2 and less so to changes in H^+ concentration.

 b. *Effect of pH:* An increase in H^+ concentration of arterial blood also stimulates pulmonary ventilation, chiefly through the peripheral (sino-aortic) chemo-receptors. Therefore, the respiratory system helps in regulation of acid–base balance of the body even when the increase in H^+ concentration is not due to CO_2 but due to non-volatile acids like sulphuric acid, phosphoric acid or lactic acid.

ROLE OF KIDNEYS

The kidneys regulate pH by either acidification or alkalinization of the urine. The renal response occurs over hours/days, and is capable of nearly complete restoration of acid–base balance.

As mentioned above, about 60 mEq of H^+ is added to the blood every day as non-volatile acids. They cannot be excreted by the lungs. They are excreted by the kidneys in an indirect manner. In the kidneys, most of the excretory products are initially filtered into the glomerular filtrate. All that is necessary for their excretion is that renal tubules reabsorb them partially or not all. In contrast, the concentration of H^+ in the blood is so small, that they cannot be excreted in this manner. Actually, most of the H^+ produced in the body do not remain as such. They are immediately buffered by HCO_3^- and other buffers. The kidney generates new hydrogen ions equivalent to the amount metabolically produced and actively secretes them into the urinary tubules, where they are buffered by phosphate and ammonium ions.

The generation of H^+ in the renal tubules is accompanied by production of HCO_3^- which diffuses into the blood circulation and replenishes the amount of HCO_3^- lost during initial buffering of the acids. In case excess of base ($NaHCO_3$) is ingested, it is excreted by the kidney by filtration followed by partial or complete non-reabsorption.

In primary pulmonary diseases such as emphysema, pulmonary excretion of CO_2 is diminished and therefore arterial pCO_2 and H^+ concentration tend to rise (respiratory acidosis). In such circumstances, renal excretion of H^+ is the only means of maintaining body pH near normal (renal compensation). Similarly in chronic renal failure, renal excretion of H^+ is diminished leading to metabolic acidosis. In such a condition, excessive loss of CO_2 by hyperventilation is the only means of maintaining body pH near normal (respiratory compensation).

Anion Gap Concept

In the plasma, total cations (Na^+, K^+, Ca^{++}, Mg^{++}, etc.) are always counter-balanced by total anions (Cl^-, HCO_3^-, PO_4^-, SO_4^-, etc). Of these ions, only Na^+, K^+, Cl^-, and HCO_3^- are routinely measured. Therefore, the concentration of *measured anions* is always less than the concentration of *measured cations*. The difference is known as the anion gap:

$$\text{Anion gap} = \{\,[Na^+] + [K^+]\,\} - \{\,[Cl^-] + [HCO_3^-]\,\}$$

Example:

Anion gap = {140 mEq/L + 4 mEq/L} − {100 mEq/L + 28 mEq/L} = 16 mEq/L

The anion gap concept is useful in the differential diagnosis of metabolic acidosis. In one group of disorders producing metabolic acidosis, the anion gap becomes larger than normal. Such disorders are said to produce *high anion gap metabolic acidosis*. In the other group of disorders, the anion gap remains normal. Such disorders are said to produce *normal anion gap metabolic acidosis* (*see* details below). *Estimation of anion gap is also a useful tool to assess mixed acid–base disorders.*

In clinical practice, since K^+ concentration does not vary grossly, the anion gap is usually calculated as follows:

$$\text{Anion gap} = [Na^+] - \{ [Cl^-] + [HCO_3^-] \}$$

Calculated in this way, the normal anion gap is 12 ± 4 mEq/L.

PATHOPHYSIOLOGY OF ACID–BASE DISORDERS

1. METABOLIC ACIDOSIS (MA)

The primary abnormality in metabolic acidosis is a decline in plasma HCO_3^- concentration. This metabolic abnormality may arise because of:

a. Increased H^+ load on the body in the form of lactic acidosis, ketoacidosis or ammonium chloride administration.
b. Deficient renal H^+ excretion.
c. Loss of HCO_3^- from GI tract or kidneys.

Metabolic acidosis may be classified into two major groups: (i) High anion gap MA and (ii) normal anion gap (hyperchloraemic) MA.

High Anion Gap MA

There are three prominent causes of high anion gap MA:
1. **Lactacidosis**
   ➢ Circulatory shock
   ➢ Severe hypoxia
2. Ketoacidosis
   ➢ Diabetic ketoacidosis
   ➢ Alcoholic ketoacidosis
   ➢ Starvation
3. **Renal failure**
   ➢ Acute or chronic

In uncompensated stage of such MA, the acid–base picture is:

$$\downarrow pH = pK + \log \frac{\downarrow HCO_3^-}{pCO_2}$$

Acidosis stimulates central and peripheral chemoreceptors causing hyperventilation (respiratory compensation). The renal compensation consists of excretion of highly acidic urine ($\uparrow H^+$ excretion). Renal compensation is not possible if MA is due to renal failure.

The respiratory compensation decreases the arterial pCO_2, whereas renal compensation generates HCO_3^- (a side effect of H^+ secretion), which partially restores the depleted HCO_3^-. The acid–base status of a case of compensated MA is as follows:

$$pH = pK + \log \frac{\downarrow HCO_3^-}{\downarrow pCO_2}$$

The two most important causes of high anion gap MA in clinical practice are diabetic ketoacidosis and renal failure. The two disorders can be differentiated by the study of serum K^+ level, which is elevated in renal failure and subnormal in diabetic ketoacidosis. A typical pattern of acid–base status and electrolyte status of patients of these two types of disorders is given below:

	Diabetic	*Uremic*
Na⁺ (mEq/L)	125	135
K⁺ (mEq/L)	3.5	5.4
HCO₃⁻ (mEq/L)	5	12
Cl⁻ (mEq/L)	90	101
pH	7.01	7.32
pCO₂ (mmHg)	20	24

Normal Anion Gap (Hyperchloremic) MA

➤ Diarrhea
➤ Renal tubular acidosis

High anion gap MA is characterized by a decrease in plasma HCO_3^- level, but no significant change in plasma Cl^- level. In hyperchloraemic type of MA, a decrease in plasma HCO_3^- is accompanied by a significant increase in plasma Cl^- and hence the name hyperchloraemic. This type of MA is typically seen in patients suffering from diarrhea or renal tubular acidosis (RTA). In diarrhea HCO_3^- is lost from the gut in exchange for Cl^-. In RTA, the failure of bicarbonate reabsorption from the renal tubules results in greater reabsorption of Cl^-. In either case, plasma Cl^- level is significantly elevated. A typical pattern of acid–base status and electrolyte pattern in a case of RTA is given below:

Na⁺ (mEq/L)	140
K⁺ (mEq/L)	2.5
HCO₃⁻ (mEq/L)	15
Cl⁻ (mEq/L)	115
pH	7.30
pCO₂ (mmHg)	30

The anion gap in the three cases with MA given above is calculated below:

$$\text{Anion gap} = [Na^+] - [(Cl^-) + (HCO_3^-)]$$

Diabetic: $125 - [90 + 5] = 30$ mEq/L (high anion gap)

Uremic : $135 - [101 + 12] = 22$ mEq/L (high anion gap)
RTA : $140 - [115 + 15] = 10$ mEq/L (normal anion gap)

2. METABOLIC ALKALOSIS

➢ Excessive sodium bicarbonate ingestion
➢ Persistent vomiting

Metabolic alkalosis occurs as a result of net gain of bicarbonate (e.g. ingestion of $NaHCO_3$ for peptic ulcer) or more often due to loss of non-volatile acids (e.g. HCl in prolonged vomiting). The primary acid–base picture in uncompensated stage is as follows:

$$\uparrow pH = pK + \log \frac{\uparrow HCO_3^-}{pCO_2}$$

For metabolic alkalosis, there is respiratory as well as renal compensation. Alkalosis inhibits the peripheral chemoreceptors, resulting in hypoventilation and elevation of pCO_2. In the kidney, metabolic alkalosis results in decreased secretion of H^+ by the renal tubules. Hence filtered bicarbonate is not completely absorbed. The urinary losses of bicarbonate decrease the extent of elevation of plasma bicarbonate. Hence the change in pH of blood is minimized. The acid–base status of a case of compensated metabolic alkalosis is as follows:

$$pH = pK + \log \frac{\uparrow HCO_3^-}{\uparrow pCO_2}$$

Metabolic alkalosis due to persistent vomiting is accompanied by not only loss of acid but also fluid from the stomach. The resulting hypovolemia becomes a strong stimulus for sodium reabsorption in the kidneys through Na^+-K^+ as well as Na^+-H^+ antiport systems. Therefore, when metabolic alkalosis is accompanied by hypovolemia, the renal response tends to aggravate alkalosis rather than correct it. It leads to hypokalemia as well. A fairly typical pattern of acid–base status and electrolytes in a patient with persistent vomiting is given below:

Na^+ (mEq/L)	140
K^+ (mEq/L)	3.2
HCO_3^- (mEq/L)	42
Cl^- (mEq/L)	84
pH	7.52
pCO_2 (mmHg)	52

3. RESPIRATORY ACIDOSIS

The primary abnormality in respiratory acidosis is elevation of $PaCO_2$ due to alveolar hypoventilation. Alveolar hypoventilation also reduces PaO_2. Therefore, hypoxemia always accompanies hypercapnea.

Acute respiratory acidosis is defined as hypercapnea developed in the time prior to renal compensation, i.e. less than 24 hours. In acute respiratory acidosis, the acid–base status is as follows:

$$\downarrow pH = pK + \log \frac{HCO_3^-}{\uparrow pCO_2}$$

Acute respiratory acidosis may be caused by:
➤ Acute airway obstruction (severe asthma)
➤ Central respiratory drive depression
  + *Drugs*: Narcotics, benzodiazepines, barbiturates
  + *Neurologic disorders*: Encephalitis, brainstem disease, trauma, poliomyelitis.
Chronic respiratory acidosis is most commonly present in
➤ Chronic obstructive pulmonary disease
  + Emphysema
  + Chronic bronchitis
➤ Chest wall deformities
  + Kyphoscoliosis

The renal compensation involves $\uparrow H^+$ excretion, as well as increased generation of HCO_3^-. The resultant increase in plasma bicarbonate concentration partially restores the blood pH towards normal:

$$pH = pK + \log \frac{\uparrow HCO_3^-}{\uparrow pCO_2}$$

Renal compensation results in elevation of plasma HCO_3^- by 3.5 mEq/L for every 10 mmHg increase in pCO_2. A fairly typical pattern of acid–base and electrolyte status of a patient with chronic respiratory acidosis is given below:

Na$^+$ (mEq/L)	137
K$^+$ (mEq/L)	4.5
HCO$_3^-$ (mEq/L)	40
Cl$^-$ (mEq/L)	90
pH	7.31
pCO$_2$ (mmHg)	75

4. RESPIRATORY ALKALOSIS

Respiratory alkalosis is the most common acid–base disorder in a critically ill patient. It is primarily caused by alveolar hyperventilation leading to decreased $paCO_2$.

$$\uparrow pH = pK + \log \frac{HCO_3^-}{\downarrow pCO_2}$$

Hypoxia due to acute pulmonary disease (e.g. pneumonia) or chronic pulmonary disease, sepsis and psychogenic hyperventilation are common causes of respiratory alkalosis.

Renal compensation to decreased arterial pCO_2 is decreased renal secretion of H^+. Consequently, bicarbonate is not generated in the kidneys. More importantly, even the filtered bicarbonate is not fully reabsorbed. Hence plasma HCO_3^- falls markedly which minimizes the change in blood pH:

$$pH = pK + \log\frac{\downarrow HCO_3^-}{\downarrow pCO_2}$$

A fairly typical pattern of acid–base and electrolytes in a patient with respiratory alkalosis is given below:

Na$^+$ (mEq/L)	135
K$^+$ (mEq/L)	3.2
HCO$_3^-$ (mEq/L)	19
Cl$^-$ (mEq/L)	105
pH	7.55
pCO$_2$ (mmHg)	22

ELECTROLYTE IMBALANCE

Electrolyte imbalance is an abnormality in the concentration of electrolytes in the body. Electrolytes play a vital role in maintaining homeostasis within the body. They help to regulate heart and neurological function, fluid balance, oxygen delivery, acid–base balance and much more. Electrolyte imbalances can develop by consuming too little or too much electrolyte as well as excreting too little or too much electrolyte. The most serious electrolyte disturbances involve abnormalities in the levels of sodium, potassium or calcium.

1. SODIUM

Hypernatraemia

Hypernatraemia means that the concentration of sodium in the blood is too high. An individual is considered to be have high sodium at levels above 145 mEq/L of sodium.

Causes
➢ Inadequate water consumption
➢ Severe dehydration
➢ Excessive loss of bodily fluids as a result of prolonged vomiting, diarrhoea, sweating, or respiratory illness
➢ Certain medications, such as diuretics and corticosteroids

Symptoms

➢ Dehydration
➢ Nausea
➢ Vomiting

➢ Fatigue
➢ Weakness
➢ Increased thirst

Hyponatremia

Hyponatremia is defined as a concentration lower than 135 mEq/L.

Causes

➤ Excessive fluid loss through the skin from sweating or burns
➤ Vomiting or diarrhoea
➤ Overhydration
➤ Congestive heart, or kidney failure
➤ Certain medications, including diuretics
➤ Syndrome of inappropriate secretion of antidiuretic hormone (SIADH)

Symptom

Severity of symptoms is directly correlated with severity of hyponatremia and rapidness of onset.

➤ Loss of appetite
➤ Nausea
➤ Vomiting
➤ Confusion

➤ Agitation
➤ Weakness
➤ Seizures, coma, and death

2. POTASSIUM

Hyperkalaemia

Hyperkalaemia means the concentration of potassium in the blood is >5 mEq/L.

Causes

➤ Kidney failure
➤ Severe acidosis, including diabetic ketoacidosis
➤ Certain medications, including some blood pressure medications and diuretics
➤ Adrenal insufficiency

Symptoms

➤ Nausea
➤ Vomiting
➤ Diarrhoea
➤ Muscle cramps
➤ Numbness
➤ Tingling
➤ Absence of reflexes
➤ Paralysis
➤ Cardiac arrhythmias that can result in death.

Hypokalaemia

Hypokalaemia is defined as the plasma concentration of potassium is <3.5 mEq/L.

Causes

➤ Severe vomiting or diarrhea
➤ Dehydration
➤ Certain medications, including laxatives, diuretics, and corticosteroids

Symptoms

➤ Muscle weakness
➤ Cramping
➤ Cardiac arrhythmias

3. CALCIUM

Hypercalcaemia

Hypercalcaemia is when plasma calcium concentration is above 10.5 mEq/dL.

Causes

➤ Hyperparathyroidism
➤ Malignancy
➤ Hyperthyroidism

➤ Excessive ingestion of vitamin D
➤ Sarcoidosis

Symptoms

➤ Abdominal pain
➤ Constipation
➤ Kidney stones

➤ Extreme thirst
➤ Excessive urination
➤ Nausea and vomiting

Hypocalcaemia

Hypocalcaemia is defined as plasma calcium level less than 9 mg/dL

Causes

➤ Vitamin D deficiency
➤ Hypoparathyroidism
➤ Multiple blood transfusions

Symptoms

➤ Muscle cramping or twitching
➤ Numbness around the mouth and fingers
➤ Arrhythmias

Basic Mechanism Involved in the Process of Inflammation and Repair

INFLAMMATION

Inflammation is the complex biological response of vascular tissues to harmful stimuli, such as pathogens, damaged cells, or irritants. Avascular tissues such as cornea, articular cartilage, intervertebral disc, etc. do not show inflammatory response. Inflammatory response is a protective attempt by the organism to remove the injurious stimuli as well as initiate the healing process. Inflammation is not a synonym for infection. Even in cases where inflammation is caused by infection, the two are not synonymous: Infection is caused by an exogenous pathogen, while inflammation is the response of the organism to the pathogen.

Inflammation can be classified as either acute or chronic. *Acute inflammation* is the initial response of the body to harmful stimuli and is achieved by the increased movement of plasma and leukocytes (initially neutrophils) from the blood into the injured tissues. A cascade of biochemical events propagates and matures the inflammatory response, involving the local vascular system, the immune system, and various cells within the injured tissue. It comes to an end within a few hours or days. Prolonged inflammation persisting for weeks or months is known as *chronic inflammation*. Whereas, neutrophil accumulation in the lesion is a hallmark of acute inflammation, chronic inflammatory lesion is characterized by the presence of lymphocytes, monocytes, macrophages and plasma cells. Another hallmark of chronic inflammation is simultaneous processes of tissue destruction and healing resulting in the formation of scar tissue. Inflammation may result from two sets of causes: Exogenous and endogenous:

A. **Exogenous factors**
   - *Mechanical injury* (traumatic injury),
   - *Physical injury* (extremely low or high temperature, ionizing irradiation, microwaves)
   - *Chemical injury* (caustic agents, poisons, venoms, etc.)
   - *Biological injury* (viruses, microorganisms, protozoan and metazoan parasites).
   - *Ischaemic injury*

B. **Endogenous factors**
   - The immunopathological responses such as *allergic* inflammations and *autoimmune* inflammatory disorders
   - Endogenous products of tissue metabolism such as gout.

<< ACUTE INFLAMMATION >>

CARDINAL SIGNS

Acute inflammation is a short-term process, usually appearing in a few minutes or hours and ceasing once the injurious stimulus has been removed. It is characterized by five cardinal signs:

➤ Redness
➤ Warmth
➤ Swelling
➤ Pain
➤ Loss of function

The first four (classical signs) were described by Celsus about 2000 years ago, while *loss of function* was added to the list later by Virchow in 1870. Redness and warmth are due to increased blood flow at body core temperature to the areas such as skin, which normally are at a lower temperature; swelling is caused by accumulation of fluid and plasma proteins in the extravascular spaces; pain is due to release of chemicals that stimulate pain nerve endings or sensitize them to other stimuli. Loss of function has multiple causes, chiefly pain and local edema.

These five signs appear when acute inflammation occurs on the body's surface. In case of acute inflammation of internal organs all the five signs may not be apparent.

ACUTE INFLAMMATORY RESPONSE

The acute inflammatory response may be discussed under two headings: (1) The vascular response and (2) The cellular response.

1. The Vascular Response

Alterations in the microvasculature (arterioles, capillaries and venules) of the injured tissue are the earliest response to the injury. It consists of: (a) hemodynamic changes and (b) changes in vascular permeability.

(a) Haemodynamic changes

Transient vasoconstriction of the arterioles and reduced blood flow is the immediate response irrespective of the type of injury. It usually lasts only a few seconds but may be prolonged up to five minutes if the injury is very severe. It is followed by:

i. Persistent and progressive vasodilatation, which begins in the arterioles and spreads to the capillaries and venules as well. This change becomes prominent within an hour of injury. Vasodilatation results in increased blood flow to the microvasculature and accounts for the clinical signs of redness and warmth. Vasodilatation is brought about by the release of vasodilator mediators by the injured tissue cells as well as by the blood cells attracted by the injury.

ii. Transudation of fluid into the extracellular space (edema) is another consequence of vasodilatation. Starling forces, chiefly capillary hydrostatic pressure and plasma protein oncotic pressure, govern the tissue fluid exchange across the capillary wall. It involves tissue fluid formation at the proximal segment of the capillary followed by reabsorption in the distal segment. Vasodilatation, by increasing the capillary hydrostatic pressure shifts the balance of the Starling forces in favor of greater exudation and decreased reabsorption. Thus, local edema results.

iii. Stasis. Loss of fluid from the capillaries leads to increased viscosity of blood flowing through the capillaries, with resultant *stasis* due to the increase in the concentration of the cells within blood. Stasis allows leukocytes to marginate along the endothelium, a process critical to their recruitment into the tissues. Normal flowing blood prevents this, as the shearing force along the periphery of the vessels moves blood cells into the middle of the vessel. Nutritional supply to the tissue may be so compromised that it may become ischemic, even necrotic.

b. Increased vascular permeability

All the blood vessels are lined by a continuous layer of endothelial cells, which provide a passive diffusion barrier. It permits free diffusion of water and solutes but restricts the movement of larger molecules such as plasma proteins and cellular components of blood. The endothelial cells are joined together by tight junctions. In inflammatory conditions, the excessive fluid transferred into extracellular space consists not only of usual water and solutes (called *transudate*), but also contains a high concentration of plasma proteins. Such a fluid is called an *exudate*. The exudate is formed because of markedly increased vascular permeability. The causes of increased vascular permeability include the following:

1. Opening of endothelial inter-cellular tight junctions, particularly in the post-capillary venules due to contraction of endothelial cells. It is mediated by release of histamine, bradykinin and other chemical mediators of inflammation. This response begins immediately after injury usually lasts for a short duration (15–30 minutes).
2. Direct injury to endothelial cells results in necrosis and appearance of physical gaps at the site of detached endothelial cells. This type of increased permeability lasts for hours or even days.
3. Endothelial injury is also mediated by leukocytes. Margination followed by leukocyte adhesion (see below) may result in activation of leukocytes. The activated leucocytes release proteolytic enzymes and toxic-free radicals which cause endothelial injury and increased vascular leakiness.
4. The capillaries, newly formed during the process of repair, are excessively leaky.

Mediators of increased vascular permeability

The primary source of vasoactive mediators of increased permeability during an inflammatory process is derived from injured tissue cells as well as plasma (Fig. 2.1).

2. The Cellular Response

Inflammatory response, which lasts more than a few hours, is characterized by accumulation of white blood cells within the area of injury. In bacterial infections, physical or thermal injury, polymorphonuclear neutrophils are first to arrive ("first line of defense"). Twenty-four to forty-eight hours later, large number of macrophages can be seen in the inflamed area. In allergic inflammation, eosinophils and mast cells predominate. In viral infections, lymphocytes are first to arrive.

A. *Polymorphonuclear neutrophils and monocyte-macrophages*

The accumulation of neutrophils and monocytes macrophages at the site of inflammation is due to the presence of locally generated chemical mediators called chemotactic factors.

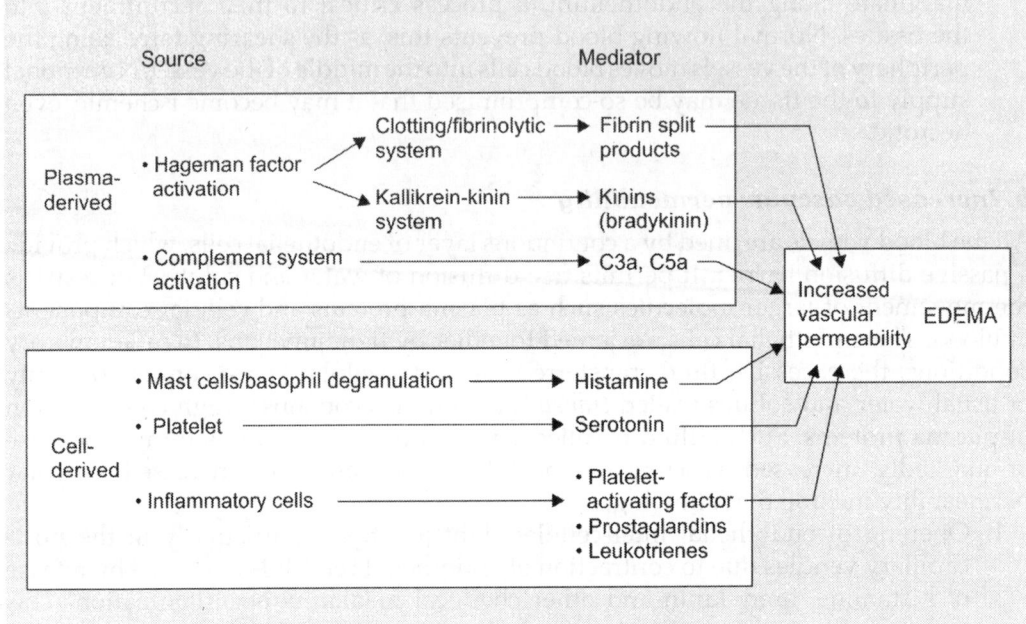

Fig. 2.1: Vasoactive mediators of increased vascular permeability during inflammation

i. **Chemotaxis:** The chemotactic-mediated transmigration of leukocytes involves initial crossing of several barriers (endothelial basement membrane and matrix), followed by transport in the interstitial fluid to the inflamed area. The process is called chemotaxis. The chemical agents which act as potent chemotactic agents include leukotrienes, platelet factor, components of complement system (C5a in particular), cytokines (IL-8 in particular), soluble bacterial products, monocyte chemo-attractant protein and eotaxin factor (for eosinophils). There is an increasing concentration gradient of chemotactic agents between an adjacent blood capillary the site of inflammation and leukocyte migration follows the gradient (Fig. 2.2).

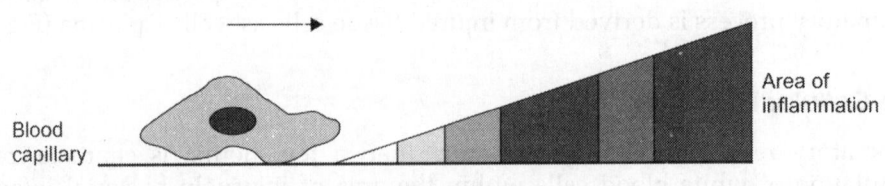

Fig. 2.2: Chemotaxis

ii. **Margination:** This is the first step towards transmigration of leukocytes out of the blood capillaries. Normal blood flow is characterized by an axial stream of red cells, leukocytes and platelets and a peripheral cell—free layer of plasma close to the vessel wall. Due to slowing of blood flow and stasis, the central stream of cells widens and blood cells including leukocytes come closer to the vessel wall. This phenomenon is known as margination.

iii. **Adhesion:** Marginated leukocytes tend to stick briefly to the endothelial cells or roll over them. Injury leads to neutralization of the normal charge on the leukocytes and endothelial cells, resulting in a loose transient adhesion of leukocytes to the endothelial cells.

iv. **Transmigration (diapedesis):** During chemotactic response, there is a characteristic change in the morphological orientation of the leukocyte (neutrophil or monocyte). It loses its classical rounded appearance and becomes wedge-shaped. At first, the leading edge passes into the space between two adjacent endothelial cells, damaging the basement membrane and passes out of the vessel wall. By amoeboid movements, rear part of the cell containing lysosomal granules and lastly the nucleus leaves the blood vessel (Fig. 2.3).

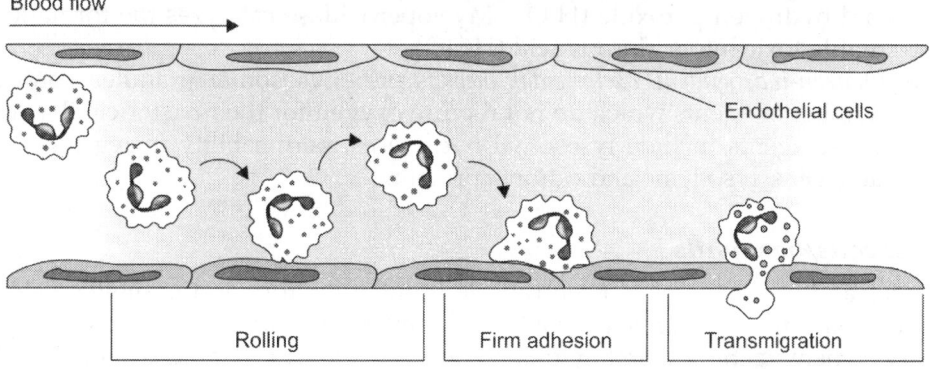

Fig. 2.3: Steps in transport of a neutrophil out of a blood capillary

v. **Phagocytosis:** Neutrophils and macrophages have an inherent capacity to recognize and engulf foreign particles. Coating of the bacteria by plasma proteins containing IgG and/or complement (opsonization) renders them more liable to phagocytosis. When a neutrophil or a macrophage becomes bound to a bacterium (or a foreign particle), there is a localized contraction of the cell under the point of contact, resulting in the formation of a cup-shaped invagination. Through the pseudopodia thrown out at the margins of the cups, the bacterium, enclosed in a vacuole, is internalized into the phagocyte and called a phagosome (Fig. 2.4). Movement of the phagosome towards the granule-rich areas of the cytoplasm results in fusion of phagosome to an adjacent lysosome. Next, the lysosomal granules are discharged into the phagosome. This phenomenon is known as *degranulation*. The lysosomal membrane is incorporated into the vacuole membrane. The resulting structure is called a phagolysosome. Generally, the release of lysosomal granules is restricted to the phagolysosome. However, when the phagosome formation occurs in a granule-rich area or the phagocyte attempts to engulf too large a particle, lysosomal granules may be discharged into extracellular space causing damage to the host tissue cells in the vicinity.

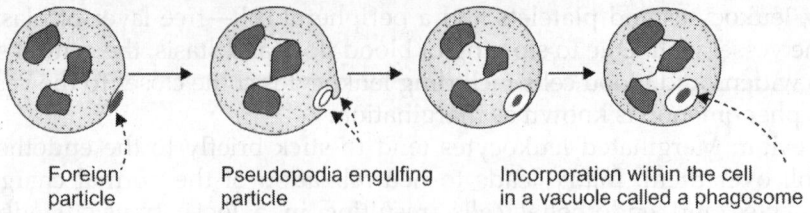

Foreign particle   Pseudopodia engulfing particle   Incorporation within the cell in a vacuole called a phagosome

Fig. 2.4: The process of phagocytosis

vi. **Bacterial killing and digestion:** This is the ultimate objective of phagocytosis. Anti-microbial agents act by the following two mechanisms:

> *Oxygen-dependent bactericidal mechanisms*: Degranulation is accompanied by activation of two enzymes present in the leukocyte granules, namely NADPH—oxidase and myeloperoxidase. Activation of NADPH-oxidase is associated with a sharp increase in oxygen consumption in the leukocyte (the respiratory burst) leading to generation of highly toxic superoxide (O_2^-) and hydrogen peroxide (H_2O_2). Myeloperoxidase catalyzes the formation of highly toxic hypochlorous acid (HClO).

> *Oxygen-independent bactericidal mechanisms*: Lysosomal granules contain a number of agents which do not require oxygen for their bactericidal activity. These agents include lysosomal hydrolases, permeability increasing factor, defensins, lysozyme and cationic protein.

B. Mast cells/basophils

Mast cells and basophils play a central role in inflammatory and immediate allergic reactions. They are able to release potent inflammatory mediators, such as histamine, proteases, chemotactic factors, cytokines and metabolites of arachidonic acid that act on the blood capillaries, smooth muscle, connective tissue, mucous glands and inflammatory cells.

Both mast cells and basophils contain special *cytoplasmic granules* which store mediators of inflammation. The extracellular release of the mediators from the mast cells (*degranulation*) may be induced by:

(a) Physical destruction, such as high temperature, mechanical trauma, ionizing irradiation, etc.;

(b) Chemical substances, such as toxins, venoms, proteases;

(c) Endogenous mediators, including tissue proteases, cationic proteins derived from eosinophils and neutrophils;

(d) Immune mechanisms which may be IgE-dependent or IgE-independent

The increase in the number of mast cells and basophils, and the enhanced secretion at sites of inflammation, can accelerate the elimination of the cause of tissue injury or, paradoxically, may lead to a chronic inflammatory response. Thus, manipulating mast-cell and basophil adhesion may be an important strategy for controlling the outcome of allergic and inflammatory responses.

C. Eosinophils

Eosinophil is a leukocyte that resides predominantly in submucosal tissue and is recruited to sites of specific immune reactions, including allergic diseases. **The**

large specific granules contain four distinct cationic proteins which exert a range of biological effects on host cells and microbial targets: *Major basic protein* (MBP), *eosinophil cationic protein* (ECP), *eosinophil-derived neurotoxin* (EDN), and *eosinophil peroxidase* (EPO). In addition, histaminase and a variety of hydrolytic lysosomal enzymes are also present in the large specific granules. These proteins have major effects not only on the potential role of eosinophils in host defense against helminthic parasites, but also in contributing to tissue dysfunction and damage in eosinophil related inflammatory and allergic diseases. Compared to neutrophils, eosinophils have limited phagocytic activity which is mainly aimed at killing multicellular parasites. Another possible beneficial function of eosinophils is the *inactivation* of mediators of anaphylaxis.

Systemic Effects of Acute Inflammation

1. Fever is due to release of interleukin 1 (a cytokine), prostaglandins or tumor necrosis factor from the inflammatory tissues, either of which can disturb the hypothalamic temperature regulating center. Fever may also be induced by certain constituents in the cell wall of dead bacteria called pyrogens.

2. Leucocytosis is a feature of infections or even non-infectious inflammations. Typically, the total leukocyte count is between 15,000 and 20,000 /μL. Usually, in bacterial infections, leucocytosis is due to neutrophilia; in viral infections due to lymphocytosis; and in allergic conditions due to eosinophilia. Some infections, e.g. typhoid fever, however, are associated with leucopoenia (neutropenia with relative lymphocytosis).

3. Lymhangitis-lymphadenitis in the lymph vessels and lymph nodes draining the area of inflammation is commonly seen. These responses represent either a non-specific reaction to chemical mediators released the inflamed tissues or an immunological response to foreign antigen.

4. Acute phase proteins. Acute inflammation is commonly accompanied by increased concentrations of several plasma proteins such as C-reactive protein, alpha-2 macroglobulin, and fibrinogen (collectively called acute phase proteins). Precise function of these proteins in inflammation is largely unclear. However, when measured in the laboratory, they can serve as useful markers of inflammation. These proteins also increase the erythrocyte sedimentation rate (ESR), a *nonspecific* indicator of inflammation. Finally, prolonged or widespread inflammation can deplete complement leading to decreased levels of certain components of complement in the serum.

5. Other symptoms such as decreased appetite, lactacidosis, negative nitrogen balance and increased slow-wave sleep are commonly seen in acute infections. Most of these seem to be produced interleukin 1.

6. Shock may develop in severe acute inflammatory conditions. Tumor necrosis factor (TNF-α), a cytokine, is one of the mediators of acute inflammation. Bacteraemia/septicaemia may result in the release of a massive amount of TNF-α leading to widespread vasodilatation and increased vascular permeability. These changes lead to intravascular volume loss, hypotension and circulatory shock. Microthrombi may be formed throughout the body which may lead to disseminated intravascular coagulation (DIC), bleeding and death.

Outcomes of Acute Inflammation

The acute inflammatory response may have one of the following four outcomes depending on whether or not injury results in significant tissue loss or the inflammatory stimulus is rapidly removed: (1) Resolution (2) healing, (3) suppuration, or (4) chronic inflammation.

1. **Resolution:** Such an outcome follows complete removal of the agent or microorganism that triggered the inflammatory response. The process includes the removal of any injured (necrotic) host cells. This is the ideal outcome for acute inflammation. It is more likely if cellular damage has been minimal, e.g. resolution of lobar pneumonia.

2. **Healing may involve two processes:**
   i. *Regeneration:* The replacement of damaged or lost tissue by normal tissue of a similar type. It occurs only in tissues that contain cells capable of dividing (e.g. epithelial tissues such as the epidermis of the skin).
   ii. *Repair: Scar formation, fibrosis.* It involves replacement of damaged or lost tissue by collagen fibers (scar tissue). This is the healing mechanism for those tissues that cannot regenerate (dermis, nerve, muscle, etc.).

3. **Suppuration and abscess formation:** If there has been a large amount of cellular necrosis, or if there is a great deal of bacterial contamination, exudates and dead leukocytes (pus) can accumulate forming an abscess. In time, connective tissue walls off the abscess and limits its spread. Resolution and healing cannot take place until adequate drainage of the abscess has been provided.

4. **Chronic inflammation:** Normally, the acute inflammatory response to cellular injury has subsided by the time tissue healing begins. If tissue destruction is prolonged, inflammation and attempts at healing occur at the same time. This produces the picture of chronic inflammation.

Mechanism of Final Resolution of Acute Inflammation

Acute inflammation normally resolves by mechanisms that have remained somewhat elusive. Emerging evidence now suggests that an active, coordinated program of resolution is initiated in the first few hours after an inflammatory response begins. After entering tissues, granulocytes promote the switch of arachidonic acid—derived prostaglandins and leukotrienes to lipoxins, which initiate the termination sequence. Neutrophil recruitment thus ceases and programmed death by apoptosis is engaged. Consequently, apoptotic neutrophils undergo phagocytosis by macrophages, leading to neutrophil clearance and release of anti-inflammatory and reparative cytokines such as transforming growth factor-β_1. The anti-inflammatory program ends with the departure of macrophages through the lymphatics.

| ALLERGIC INFLAMMATION

An allergic reaction is the result of an inappropriate immune response triggering inflammation. A common example is hay fever, which is caused by a hypersensitive response by skin mast cells to allergens. Pre-sensitized mast cells respond by degranulation, releasing vasoactive chemicals such as histamine. These chemicals propagate an excessive inflammatory response characterized by blood vessel dilation, production of pro-inflammatory molecules, cytokine release, and recruitment of leukocytes. Severe inflammatory response may mature into a systemic response known as anaphylaxis.

< CHRONIC INFLAMMATION >

Chronic inflammation occurs when the damaging stimulus persists and the process of *continuing tissue necrosis, organization, and repair all occur concurrently*. In addition to acute inflammation, the specific defences of the immune system are activated around the area of damage, and tissues are infiltrated by activated lymphoid cells.

The chronic inflammatory tissue shows:
➢ Necrotic cell debris
➢ Acute inflammatory exudate
➢ Vascular and fibrous granulation tissue
➢ Lymphoid cells
➢ Macrophages
➢ Collagenous scar

Chronic inflammation may be caused by one of the following three mechanisms:

i. **Chronic inflammation following an acute inflammation:** When tissue destruction is extensive or bacteria survive and persist at the site of inflammation, e.g. osteomyelitis or pneumonia leading to a lung abscess.

ii. **Recurrent attacks of acute inflammation:** Repeated attacks of acute inflammation may culminate in chronicity of the disease process, e.g. pyelonephritis resulting from recurrent attacks of urinary tract infection, or repeated attacks of acute cholecystitis culminating in chronic cholecystitis.

iii. **Chronic inflammation starting *de novo*:** In such cases, the inflammatory agent produces a chronic inflammatory response to begin with.

GENERAL FEATURES OF CHRONIC INFLAMMATION

Ordinarily, agents that produce an acute inflammatory response are removed by the neutrophils and macrophages by phagocytosis and digestion. However, certain agents cannot be removed by acute inflammatory response, e.g. *Mycobacterium tuberculosis*, fungus or a suture. The mechanism of dealing with such indigestible agents is termed chronic or granulomatous inflammation. Chronic inflammation response primarily serves to contain the pathological process, as well as to remove the offending agent, if possible. Though, chronic inflammatory responses may somewhat differ in detail, depending on the offending agent, the following features are common to all chronic inflammations: (A) Mononuclear cell infiltration, (B) tissue destruction and necrosis, and (C) proliferative changes.

A. Mononuclear Cell Infiltration

i. **Macrophages:** The macrophages comprise the most important cells in chronic inflammation. These cells are recruited by chemotactic migration from the circulation as well as by local proliferation. Activated macrophages release several biologically active substances such as neutral and acid proteases, oxygen-derived reactive metabolites and cytokines. These agents bring about tissue destruction, neo-vascularization and fibrosis. Chronic inflammatory lesions usually show some other chronic inflammatory cells:

ii. **Lymphocytes:** These cells are a prominent feature of chronic inflammatory lesion. They perform vital functions both in cell-mediated and humoral immune responses. The T-lymphocytes function not only as cytotoxic killer cells but also regulate macrophage recruitment and activation through secretion of lymphokines (cytokines) and modulate antibody production.

iii. **Plasma cells:** These cells are also usually present in a chronic inflammatory lesion. Plasma cells are immune-activated B-lymphocytes rich in cytoplasmic reticulum. These cells are the primary source of antibodies specific to the antigen present at the site of chronic lesion.

B. Tissue Destruction

It is one of the important features of most of the chronic inflammatory responses. As mentioned above, it is brought about by several biologically active substances released by activated macrophages.

C. Proliferative Changes

As a result of necrosis, proliferation of small blood vessels is stimulated. Eventually, collagen is laid down and healing by fibrosis occurs (Fig. 2.5).

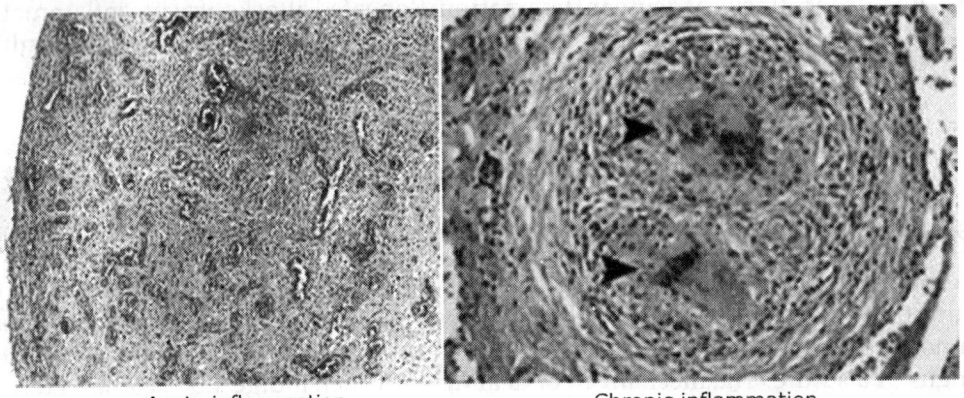

Acute inflammation   Chronic inflammation

Fig. 2.5: Histological appearance of acute and chronic inflammation

Table 2.1: Summary of differences between acute and chronic inflammation

Acute inflammation	Chronic inflammation
Abrupt injury	Persistent injury
Onset is well-defined	Vague onset
Prominent symptoms	Symptoms often subdued, and /or insidious
Prominent vascular effects and exudate	Mild tissue effects
Exudate rich in neutrophils	Exudate rich in lymphocytes and macrophages
Connective tissue proliferation occurs after inflammation subsides.	Connective tissue proliferation is concurrent with on-going inflammation.

BASIC PRINCIPLES OF WOUND HEALING

If there is an injury to the skin, under normal circumstances, the wound heals in a few days. The process of wound healing consists of four overlapping phases:

1. **Haemostasis phase:** Injury to the skin or other tissues results in bleeding. The first step in wound healing involves stoppage of bleeding (haemostasis). Haemostasis starts when blood leaks out of the body. The circulating platelets collect at the site of injury, stick together, form platelet plug and seal the break in the wall of the blood vessel. This step is known as primary haemostasis. However, the platelet is soft and temporary. In the next step known as secondary haemostasis, the blood collected at the site of injury clots. Clotting of blood seals the leak in blood vessels permanently. The blood clot reinforces the platelet plug with threads of fibrin which are like a molecular binding agent. The hemostasis stage of wound healing happens within a few minutes.

2. **Inflammatory phase:** Inflammation is the second stage of wound healing and begins right after the injury when the injured blood vessels lose blood. Inflammation both controls bleeding and prevents infection. The acute inflammatory response has been described in detail earlier in this chapter. During the inflammatory phase, damaged cells are removed from the wound area. Swelling, heat, pain and redness commonly seen during this stage of wound healing are signs of acute inflammation. If some bacteria get into the wound, blood macrophages remove the pathogens. Inflammation is a natural part of the wound healing process and only problematic if prolonged or excessive, if infection cannot be controlled.

3. **Proliferative phase:** The proliferative phase features three distinct stages:
   1. Filling the wound
   2. Contraction of the wound margins
   3. Covering the wound by epithelialization

   The gap in the skin is filled by newly built tissue consisting of collagen fibres and extracellular matrix. In addition, a new network of blood vessels grows into the wound bed forming shiny, deep red granulation tissue. When tissues are injured, fibroblasts around the injured region differentiate into myofibroblasts, a type of highly contractile cells that produce abundant extracellular matrix proteins. It has become clear that both fibroblasts and myofibroblasts play a critical role in the wound healing process. Fibroblast cells lay down collagen fibers. Myofibroblasts cause the wound to contract by gripping the wound edges and pulling them together. In healthy stages of wound healing, granulation tissue is pink or red and uneven in texture. Moreover, healthy granulation tissue does not bleed easily. Dark granulation tissue can be a sign of infection, ischemia, or poor perfusion. In the final phase of the proliferative stage of wound healing, epithelial cells resurface the injury. It is important to remember that epithelialization happens faster when wounds are kept moist and hydrated (Fig. 2.6).

4. **Maturation phase:** When collagen is laid down during the proliferative phase, it is disorganized and the wound is thick. During the maturation phase, collagen is aligned along tension lines and water is reabsorbed so the collagen fibers can lie closer together and cross-link. Cross-linking of collagen reduces scar thickness and also makes the skin area of the wound stronger. When the wound fully closes, the cells that had been used to repair the wound but which are no longer

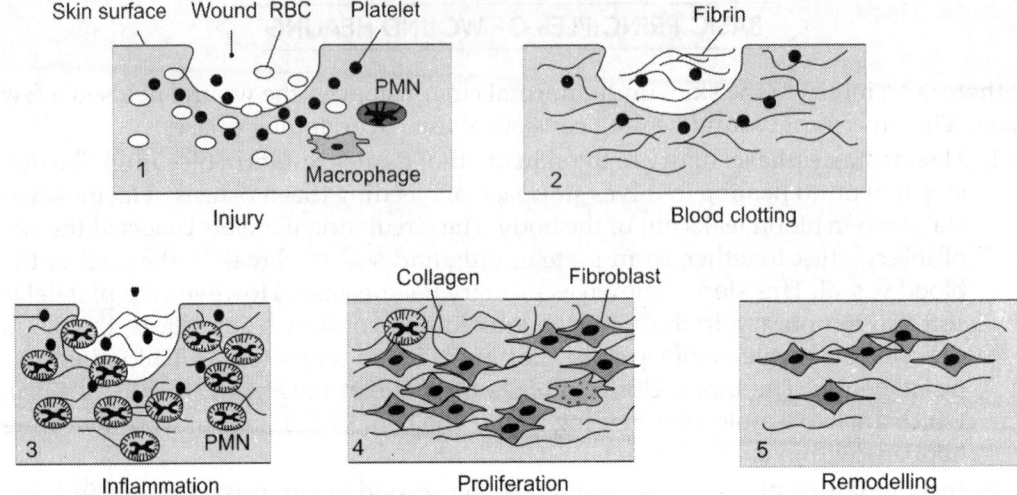

Fig. 2.6: Stages of wound healing

needed are removed by apoptosis. Generally, remodelling begins about 21 days after an injury and can continue for a year or more.

The stages of wound healing are a complex and fragile process. Failure to progress in the stages of wound healing can lead to chronic wounds. Factors that lead up to chronic wounds include venous disease, infection, diabetes, poor nutrition, old age, etc.

SCAR

A scar is an area of fibrous tissue that replaces normal skin after an injury. Scars result from the biological process of wound repair in the skin, as well as in other organs and tissues of the body. Thus, scarring is a natural part of the healing process (Fig. 2.7).

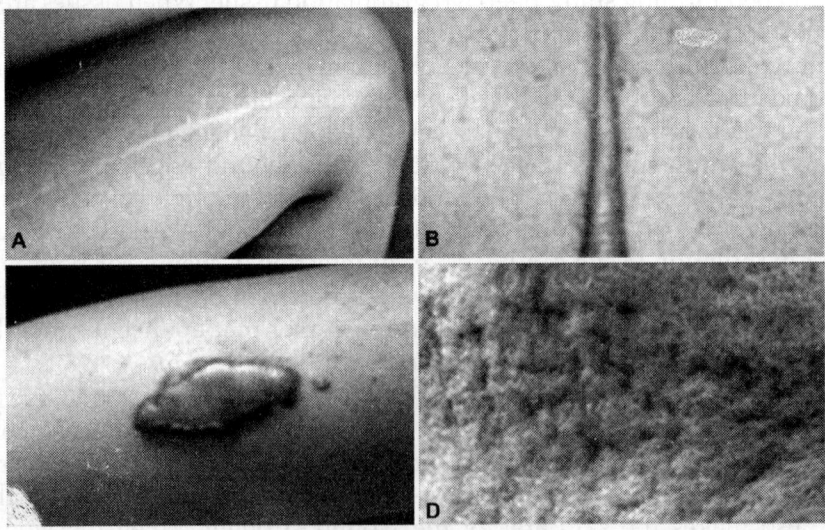

Fig. 2.7: Types of scar. (A) Normal; (B) hypertrophic; (C) keloid; (D) atrophic

With the exception of very minor lesions, every wound (e.g. after accident, disease, or surgery) results in some degree of scarring.

Hypertrophic scars occur when the body overproduces collagen, which causes the scar to be raised above the surrounding skin. Hypertrophic scars take the form of a red raised lump on the skin. They usually occur within 4 to 8 weeks following wound infection or wound closure with excess tension and/or other traumatic skin injuries.

Keloid scars are a more serious form of excessive scarring, because they can grow indefinitely into large, itchy tumorous mass. Keloids differ from normal mature scars in type of collagen and size. Some people are prone to keloid formation and may develop them in several places.

Atrophic scars takes the form of a sunken recess in the skin, which has a pitted appearance. These are caused when underlying structures supporting the skin, such as fat or muscle, are lost. This type of scarring is often associated with acne or chickenpox.

Disorder of
Cardiovascular System

◁ HYPERTENSION ▷

Hypertension is a serious medical condition that significantly increases the risks of heart, brain, kidney and other diseases. According to WHO, in 2015, worldwide 25% of males and 20% of females were suffering from hypertension. Of these, only 20% of patients had BP under control. In India about 33% urban and 25% rural population is hypertensive. More worrying is the report that only one-tenth of rural and one-fifth of urban Indian hypertensive population have their BP under control. Hypertension is directly responsible for 57% of all stroke deaths and 24% of all coronary heart disease deaths in India.

Definition

Hypertension is defined as arterial blood pressure greater than 140 mmHg and/or diastolic pressure greater than 90 mmHg. Systolic pressure 120–140 mmHg or diastolic pressure 80–90 mmHg is known as prehypertension. In a vast majority of cases of hypertension, no definite cause can be detected. Such patients are said to suffer from "**essential hypertension.**" In a small percentage of patients of hypertension, a definite cause can be found, such as kidney disease or/and endocrine disorder. Such cases are said to suffer from **secondary hypertension.**

Symptoms

In most of the cases of high blood pressure, there are no symptoms till the complications occur. When blood pressure is very high, severe headache may be reported.

| AETIOLOGY AND PATHOGENESIS OF ESSENTIAL HYPERTENSION

Blood pressure = Cardiac output × Peripheral resistance

= CO × PR

Regardless of the origin of hypertension, the actual increase in arterial blood pressure is caused by either an increase in peripheral vascular resistance (PR) or an increase in cardiac output (CO). The former is determined by the vascular tone (i.e.

state of constriction) of systemic resistance vessels, whereas the latter is determined by heart rate and stroke volume. In later stages of hypertension, only peripheral resistance is found to be increased; CO is normal. However, as discussed below, in early stages of hypertension, many individuals have increased sympathetic activity leading to increased CO.

1. Genetic Predisposition

Epidemiological studies have shown the importance of genetic predisposition in the development of essential hypertension. If family history of hypertension is present, the subject has 3–4 fold greater chance of developing hypertension, at an age earlier than general population. Although genetics appears to contribute to essential hypertension, the exact mechanism has not been established. Genetic factors interact with environmental factors such as high salt intake, male sex, smoking, obesity, stress and physical inactivity, etc.

2. Sympathetic Overactivity

There is evidence for a widespread autonomic abnormality in the early phases of hypertension. Overwhelming and excessive sympathetic activity is consistently present in some patients since their childhood. In early stages of hypertension, blood pressure is elevated when recorded in doctor's clinic, but found to be normal when recorded at home. Such cases are said to suffer from "white coat hypertension". Earlier, it was believed that persons with "white coat hypertension" do not develop established hypertension. There is no support for such an assertion; in fact, such patients are at a high risk of future accelerated hypertension. The hallmark of the sympathetic over-activity in these patients is the so-called hyperkinetic state that is best characterized by borderline elevation of blood pressure, a fast heart rate and an increased cardiac output even at rest.

Both the hyperkinetic state and sympathetic overactivity are less readily recognizable later in the course of hypertension. A large proportion of previously hyperkinetic patients later develop established hypertension. It is not clear how from a fast heart rate/high cardiac output form of borderline hypertension is transformed later into the normal cardiac output/high vascular resistance profile that is characteristic of established hypertension.

3. Role of Sodium Intake

Essential hypertension is seen primarily in societies with average sodium intake above 100 mEq/day (2.3 g sodium); it is rare in societies with average sodium intakes of less than 50 mEq/day (1.2 g sodium). These epidemiological observations led to the suggestion that the development of hypertension requires a threshold level of sodium intake. This factor effect appears to be independent of other risk factors for hypertension, such as obesity.

4. Vascular Hyper-reactivity

Hypertensive patients manifest greater vasoconstrictive response to infused norepinephrine or immersion of one hand in ice-cold water (cold pressor test) than normal individuals. Greater vasoconstrictive response to norepinephrine has also been demonstrated in normotensive offspring of hypertensive patients as compared to controls with no family history of hypertension. It suggests that vascular hyper-reactivity may be genetic in origin.

5. Renin-angiotensin-aldosterone-system (RAAS)

In patients of essential hypertension, about 15% have mildly elevated plasma renin activity. In another 60% of hypertensives, plasma renin activity is "within the normal range" but it may inappropriate in presence of elevated blood pressure. Less than 25% patients of essential hypertension have subnormal plasma renin activity. Moreover, favorable therapeutic response to RAAS blockers suggests that renin-dependent mechanism may be involved in the pathogenesis in about 70% cases of essential hypertension. The fundamental cause of elevated renin activity in such cases is not yet clear. It could be due to a chronic sympathetic overactivity. This possibility is supported by the reports that administration of β-blockers in cases with essential hypertension leads to a decrease in plasma renin activity paralleled by a decrease in arterial blood pressure.

6. Endothelial dysfunction

Due to its position between blood stream and vascular smooth muscle, endothelial dysfunction could either be a consequence or a causative factor in essential hypertension. In recent years, considerable evidence has suggested that changes in vascular endothelial function may cause the increase in vascular tone. For example, in hypertensive patients, the vascular endothelium produces less nitric oxide (intrinsic vasodilator). Moreover, the vascular smooth muscle is less sensitive to the actions of this powerful vasodilator. There may also be an increase in endothelin (a vasoconstrictor) production by the endothelial cells, which can enhance vasoconstrictor tone.

COMPLICATIONS OF UNTREATED ESSENTIAL HYPERTENSION

1. Atherosclerosis

Many of the complications of hypertension are related to the effects of sustained elevations of blood pressure on vasculature and heart. Atherosclerosis is commonly associated with and is accelerated by long-standing hypertension. Most of the adverse outcomes in hypertension are associated with thrombosis rather than bleeding. Atherosclerosis predisposes the hypertensive patient to coronary thrombosis and cerebral stroke. Cerebral strokes are more often due to thrombosis rather than hemorrhage in the cerebral vessels. The excess morbidity and mortality related to hypertension are progressive over the whole range of systolic and diastolic blood pressures, and not limited to high values only. However, target-organ damage varies markedly between individuals with similar levels of hypertension. Atherosclerosis may also result in aortic aneurysm or peripheral arterial disease.

2. Hypertensive Cardiomyopathy

Sustained increase in blood pressure (afterload) results in *hypertrophy and subsequent dilatation* of left ventricle (Fig. 1.10). Electrocardiographic evidence of left ventricular hypertrophy is found in up to 15% of persons with chronic hypertension. Left ventricular hypertrophy may cause or facilitate many cardiac complications of hypertension, including myocardial ischemia, congestive heart failure, ventricular arrhythmias.

➤ **Cerebrovascular complications:** Hypertension is an important risk factor for cerebral stroke. Approximately 85% of strokes are due to thrombosis and the remainder are due to hemorrhage in cerebral blood vessels.

The term *hypertensive encephalopathy* is used to describe a group of symptoms and signs that *sometimes* follow a sudden and sustained rise of blood pressure. The symptoms are characterized by a severe headache, restless, impaired judgment and memory, confusion, somnolence and stupor. If the condition is not treated, these neurological symptoms may worsen and ultimately turn into a coma. Cerebral encephalopathy seems to result from a failure of autoregulation of cerebral blood flow. The autoregulation seems to fail when hypertension becomes excessive.

➤ **Retinopathy:** The primary response of the retinal arterioles to systemic hypertension is vasoconstriction. However, sustained hypertension leads to disruption of the blood—retinal barrier, increased vascular permeability and secondary arteriolosclerosis. Loss of vision may occur.

➤ **Renal complications:** Renal failure is one of the important complications of chronic hypertension. Sustained elevation of blood pressure damages renal microvasculature. Renal damage itself is a cause of hypertension (see secondary hypertension below), starting a vicious cycle.

➤ **Sexual dysfunction:** Sexual dysfunction is more common and more severe in men with hypertension than it is in the general population. Hypertension is itself the major cause of erectile dysfunction. Experimental studies indicate that essential hypertension results in structural and functional changes in penile vasculature. Cavernous vessels are affected by chronic elevation of arterial blood pressure in the same fashion as other blood vessels. Marked hypertrophy in the smooth muscle of cavernous vessels, increased smooth muscle layer in cavernous space and increased extracellular matrix (collagen) explain the pathophysiological mechanism of erectile dysfunction in essential hypertension.

PATHOPHYSIOLOGICAL BASIS OF TREATMENT OF ESSENTIAL HYPERTENSION

Non-pharmacological Measures

➤ Reduction or elimination of factors such as stress, smoking, obesity
➤ Regular aerobic exercise
➤ Restriction of dietary calories, salt, cholesterol, and saturated fats

Pharmacological Measures

A variety of drugs are being used in the treatment of essential hypertension. They reduce cardiac output, peripheral resistance or both (Fig. 3.1).

Secondary Hypertension

Secondary hypertension is defined as hypertension which is caused by an underlying well-defined primary cause. It is much less common than the essential hypertension, affecting only 5% of hypertensive patients. Some of the causes of secondary hypertension are treatable.

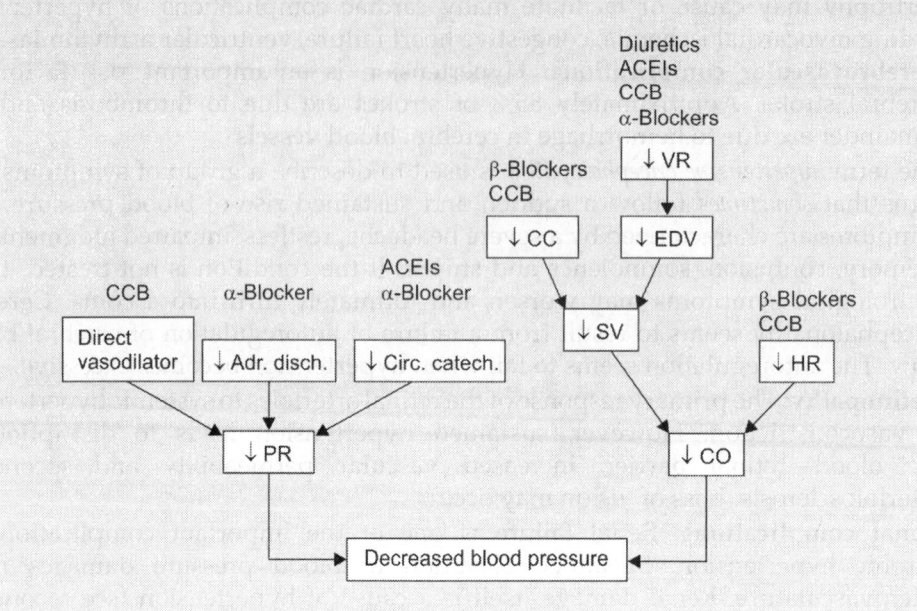

Fig. 3.1: Mechanism of action of anti-hypertensive drugs. (CC = Cardiac contractility; VR = Venous return; SV = Stroke volume; EDV = End-diastolic volume; HR = Heart rate; PR = Peripheral resistance; CO = Cardiac output; CCB = Calcium channel blockers; ACEIs = Angiotensin converting enzyme inhibitors).

Symptoms

Like primary hypertension, secondary hypertension usually has no specific signs or symptoms, even if blood pressure has reached dangerously high levels.

Causes

➢ **Chronic kidney disease** (chronic glomerulonephritis)
➢ **Renal artery stenosis**
➢ **Cushing syndrome** (increased secretion of cortisol by a tumor of adrenal cortex).
➢ **Aldosteronism** (increased secretion of aldosterone by a tumor of adrenal cortex).
➢ **Pheochromocytoma** (increased secretion norepinephrine and epinephrine by a tumor of adrenal medulla).
➢ **Coarctation of the aorta:** There is congenital narrowing (coarctation) in the thoracic aorta. Hypertension is recorded in upper part of the body only.

ATHEROSCLEROSIS

Arteriosclerosis is the thickening, hardening, and loss of elasticity of the walls of arteries. This process gradually restricts the blood flow to one's organs and tissues and can lead to severe organ damage. **Atherosclerosis,** which is a specific form of arteriosclerosis, is caused by the build up of fatty acid-cholesterol plaques in the artery walls.

ATHEROSCLEROSIS

Atherosclerosis develops primarily in large elastic arteries, e.g. aorta and carotid artery, or large or medium-sized muscular arteries such as coronary, cerebral, renal and popliteal arteries. Atherosclerosis can lead to serious complications such as coronary artery disease, cerebral stroke, peripheral arterial disease (gangrene of feet or legs).

Risk factors associated with atherosclerosis, including:

➤ Elevated blood cholesterol and triglyceride levels
➤ High blood pressure   ➤ Obesity
➤ Smoking   ➤ Physical inactivity
➤ Diabetes mellitus

Symptoms

Atherosclerosis develops gradually. Mild atherosclerosis usually does not have any symptoms. Symptoms develop only when narrowing of the artery is so severe that adequate amount of blood does not reach the tissues or organs. At that time symptoms depend on the artery affected.

➤ **Coronary artery:** Symptoms of angina or myocardial infarction
➤ **Cerebral artery:** Symptoms of cerebral stroke.
➤ **Renal artery:** Development of hypertension or symptoms of renal failure.
➤ **Popliteal artery:** Pain in the legs while walking (claudication)

Pathogenesis of Atherosclerosis

Aetiological factors named above induce hypercholesterolemia, which disturbs vascular homeostasis, including a decrease in nitrous oxide bioactivity, an increase in superoxide production, an increase in adhesion molecules and attenuation of endothelium-dependent vasodilatation.

The earliest pathologic lesion of atherosclerosis is the fatty streak. The fatty streak is the result of focal accumulation of serum lipoproteins within the intima of the vessel wall. Gradually, the fatty streak progress to form a fibrous plaque (Fig. 3.2).

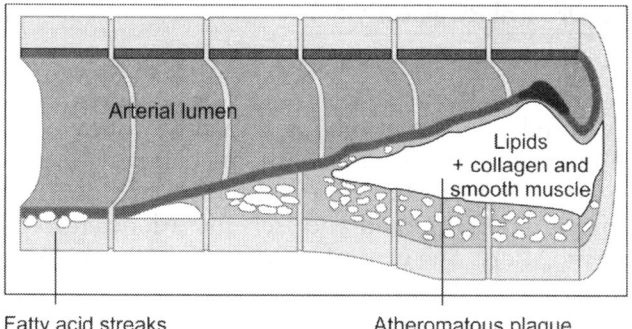

Fig. 3.2: Pathogenesis of atheromatous plaque

Circulating monocytes infiltrate the intima of the vessel wall. The combination of diabetes and hypertension appears to have an additive effect on monocyte adhesion. These tissue macrophages act as scavenger cells, taking up LDL cholesterol and forming the characteristic foam cell of early atherosclerosis. These activated macrophages produce numerous factors that are injurious to the endothelium. Atherosclerotic plaque is the result of progressive lipid accumulation along with migration and proliferation of smooth muscle cells. Growth of the fibrous plaque results in progressive luminal narrowing.

Microscopy reveals lipid-laden macrophages, T-lymphocytes and smooth muscle cells in varying proportions. Atheromatous plaques convert the smooth lining of tunica intima of the blood vessels to roughened surface (Fig. 3.3) prone to thrombosis. Moreover, developing atherosclerotic plaques are prone to necrosis. Loss of the overlying endothelium or rupture of the protective fibrous cap may result in exposure of the thrombogenic contents of the core of the plaque to the circulating blood. This exposure constitutes an advanced or complicated lesion. A plaque rupture may result in thrombus formation leading to partial or complete occlusion of the blood vessel.

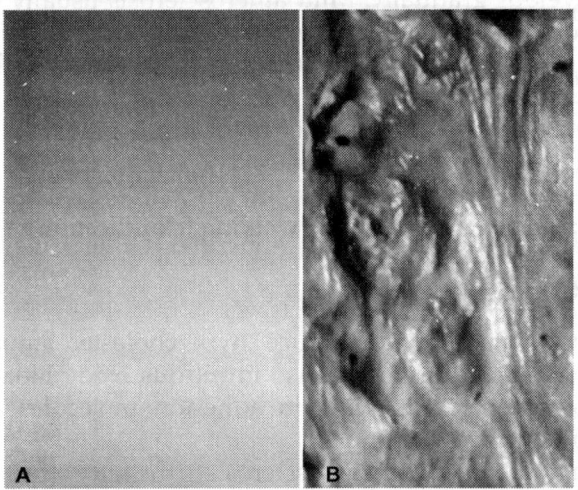

Fig. 3.3: Aorta (A) Smooth inner surface; (B) atheromatous inner surface

| COMPLICATIONS OF ATHEROSCLEROSIS

Thrombosis

Rupture of plaque is followed by thrombus formation (intravascular clotting). The rough endothelial lining of a blood vessel attracts platelet adhesion and activation. Activated platelets result in formation of an intravascular clot. The **thrombus** results in critical narrowing of arterial lumen and ischemia (deficient blood supply) in the tissues supplied by the artery. The clinical response to ischemia caused by obstructive atherosclerosis is dependent on the artery involved:

Artery involved	Disease produced
Coronary artery	Myocardial ischemia/infarction
Carotid artery	Cerebral stroke
Renal artery	Renal failure
Popliteal artery	Gangrene of lower limbs

CORONARY ARTERY DISEASE

Cardiovascular diseases are the number 1 cause of death globally. An estimated 17.9 million people died from CVDs in 2016, representing 31% of all global deaths. Of these deaths, 85% are due to heart attack and stroke. In India, studies have reported increasing prevalence of coronary artery disease over the last 60 years, from 1% to 9–10% in urban populations and <1% to 4–6% in rural populations.

▌MYOCARDIAL OXYGEN SUPPLY

The myocardial oxygen supply depends on: (i) Oxygen content of the arterial blood, and (ii) the rate of coronary blood flow. The oxygen content of arterial blood may be decreased because of decreased hemoglobin concentration or because of poor systemic blood oxygenation (hypoxic hypoxia). Thus, angina may be a presenting feature of a patient with severe anemia or lung disease. In the absence of anemia or lung disease, oxygen supply to the heart is determined by rate of coronary blood flow.

In most other organs, because of greater pressure head, blood flow is greater during systole than in diastole of the heart. However, in case of myocardium, the reverse is true. The coronary arteries that run on the surface of the heart are called epicardial coronary arteries. Branches of epicardial arteries run into and supply blood to the myocardium are called subendocardial coronary vessels. During systole, myocardial contraction has a strangulating effect on the blood vessels passing through the cardiac muscle fibers. Because of this, blood flow in the subendocardial vessels stops. As a result, most myocardial perfusion occurs during diastole when the subendocardial coronary vessels are patent because of absence of extramural pressure (Fig. 3.4A).

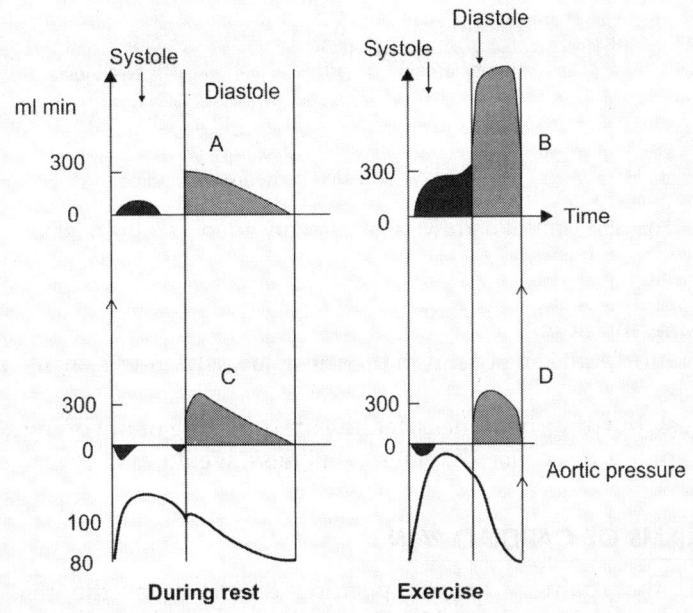

Fig. 3.4: Left coronary blood flow in systole and diastole at rest and during exercise. **(A, B)** Normal healthy person; **(C, D)** a patient with coronary artery disease.

Although coronary vessels are supplied with sympathetic and parasympathetic nerve fibers, the coronary vascular resistance is chiefly determined by intrinsic metabolic factors rather than neural control. Local vasodilator metabolites such as adenosine (chiefly) and other products of anoxic metabolism (lactate, H^+, certain prostaglandins) regulate coronary blood flow by a direct action on vascular smooth muscle. During exercise, greater release of local vasodilator metabolites assures greater blood flow in the coronary arteries (Fig. 3.4B)

Atherosclerotic narrowing of coronary arteries produces its effects mainly by hypo-perfusion (decreased blood supply) of the myocardium. The effect may range from angina to myocardial infarction.

ANGINA PECTORIS

In normal individuals during exercise, by the local metabolite control, coronary arteriolar resistance decreases in proportion to the increase in O_2 demand of the myocardium. Thus, coronary blood flow increases in proportion to the oxygen demand of myocardium. (Fig. 3.4A and B). When atherosclerotic narrowing is greater than 60–70%, (Fig. 3.5), coronary blood flow cannot increase during exercise in spite of presence of vasodilator metabolites (Fig. 3.4C and D). Therefore, myocardial ischemia results; which is commonly intermittent (only during exertion). Anginal pain is characterized by the fact that it occurs only at times of increased myocardial oxygen demand such as exertion or emotional excitement, but subsides by rest. Such a condition is known as *angina*. In angina, pain may be localized to substernum or referred to left arm, neck, jaw (Fig. 3.6).

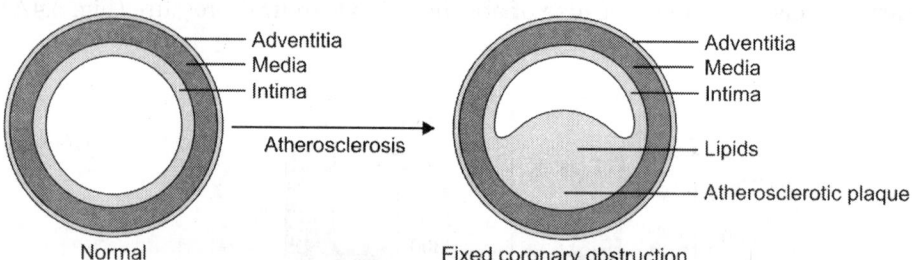

Fig. 3.5: Critical narrowing of coronary artery causing angina

Symptoms

Angina symptoms include:
➤ Pain or discomfort that can spread to the chest, jaw, shoulders, arms (mostly the left arm) and back.
➤ Chest tightness, burning, heaviness, feeling of squeezing or not being able to breathe.
➤ Angina will sometimes cause dizziness, paleness, weakness.

THE MECHANISMS OF CARDIAC PAIN

It is presumed that pain of angina pectoris results from the release of anoxic metabolites (adenosine, bradykinin) by the myocardium. These metabolites excite the sensory ends of the sympathetic and vagal afferent fibers supplying the heart. Within the spinal cord, cardiac sympathetic afferent impulses may converge with impulses from somatic thoracic structures, which may be the basis for referred cardiac pain, for example, to the left arm.

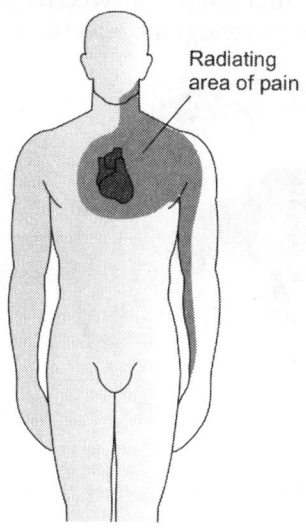

Fig. 3.6: Location of pain in angina

PATHOPHYSIOLOGIC BASIS OF TREATMENT OF ANGINA

For the immediate relief of angina pain, the patient is advised to take a sublingual tablet of nitroglycerin.

Nitroglycerin is converted to a powerful vasodilator nitric oxide (NO) in the body. It may produce some dilation of coronary arteries, but the major action is venous vasodilation. Venodilation causes pooling of blood within the venous system, reducing preload to the heart. This causes a decrease in cardiac work, and cardiac oxygen demand and hence relieves angina pain.

MYOCARDIAL INFARCTION

When the myocardial ischaemia progresses to a degree that irreversible necrosis of a part of myocardium occurs, an acute myocardial infarction (MI) is said to have occurred. An acute MI almost always results from an acute thrombotic obstruction of an atherosclerotic coronary artery (Fig. 3.7).

Symptoms

➤ Chest pain or discomfort, possibly described as pressure, squeezing, burning or fullness
➤ Pain in left arm, neck, jaw, shoulder or back accompanying chest pain
➤ Nausea
➤ Fatigue
➤ Shortness of breath
➤ Sweating
➤ Dizziness

In acute MI, the pain has same characteristics as angina, but it is far more severe, lasts longer, may radiate more widely, and not relieved by rest or nitroglycerin. Pain may be due to accumulation of anoxic metabolites as well as products of tissue necrosis. The pain is accompanied by greater psychogenic effects, i.e. feeling of impending death.

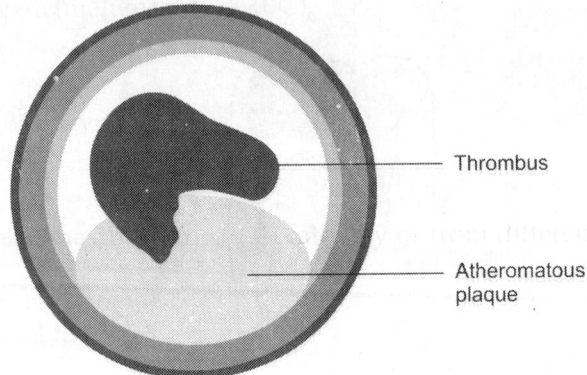

Fig. 3.7: Coronary thrombosis over atherosclerotic plaque

Pathogenesis

Acute myocardial infarction (MI) indicates irreversible myocardial injury resulting in necrosis of a significant portion of myocardium (generally >1 cm). Myocardial infarction is usually due to thrombotic occlusion of a coronary vessel caused by rupture of a vulnerable plaque. Ischemia induces profound metabolic and ionic perturbations in the affected myocardium. Prolonged myocardial ischemia results in ischemic necrosis of the myocardium (Fig. 3.8). The adult mammalian heart has negligible regenerative capacity, thus the infarcted myocardium heals through formation of a scar (Fig. 3.9). Infarct healing is intertwined with geometric remodelling of the chamber, characterized by dilation, hypertrophy of viable segments, and progressive dysfunction.

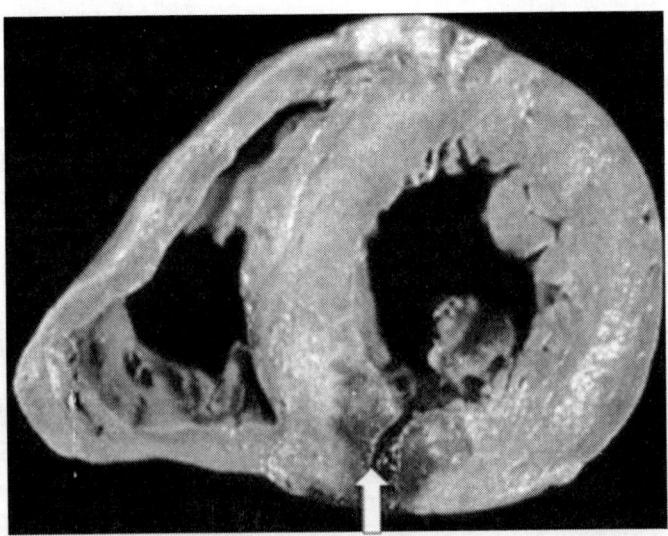

Fig. 3.8: Myocardial infarction (arrow)

Cell membrane damage in acute MI leads to release of certain intracellular enzymes. Increase in their plasma levels is used as a diagnostic evidence of myocardial infarction.

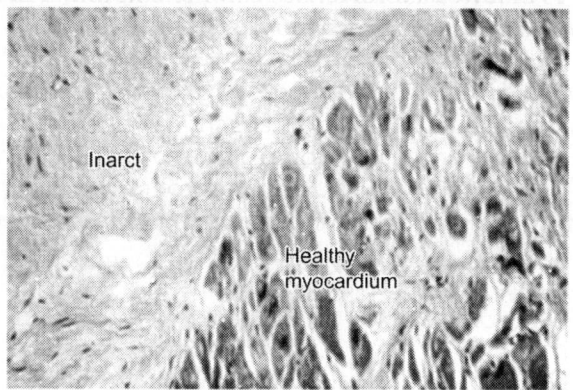

Fig. 3.9: Histology of myocardial infarct

Risk Factors

➢ **Age:** Men age 45 or older and women age 55 or older are more likely to have a heart attack than are younger men and women.
➢ **Tobacco:** This includes smoking and long-term exposure to second-hand smoke.
➢ **High blood pressure:** Over time, high blood pressure can damage coronary arteries.
➢ **High blood cholesterol or triglyceride levels:** A high level of low-density lipoprotein (LDL) cholesterol (the 'bad' cholesterol) is most likely to narrow arteries. A high level of triglycerides, a type of blood fat related to your diet, also ups your risk of heart attack.
➢ **Obesity:** Obesity is associated with high blood cholesterol levels, high triglyceride levels, high blood pressure and diabetes.
➢ **Diabetes.**
➢ **Family history of heart attack**
➢ **Lack of physical activity**
➢ **Stress.**

Diagnosis

1. **Electrocardiogram:** An electrocardiogram (ECG) is a recording of the electrical activity of the heart. Abnormalities in the electrical activity usually occur with heart attacks and can identify the areas of heart muscle that are deprived of oxygen and/or areas of muscle that have died (Fig. 3.10). In a patient with typical symptoms of heart attack (such as crushing chest pain) and characteristic changes of heart attack on the ECG, a secure diagnosis of heart attack can be made quickly in the emergency room and treatment can be started immediately.
2. **Blood tests:** Cardiac enzymes are proteins that are released into the blood by dying heart muscles. These cardiac enzymes are creatine kinase (CK-MB), and troponin, and their levels can be measured in blood (Fig. 3.11). These cardiac enzymes typically are elevated in the blood several hours after the onset of a heart attack. Currently, troponin levels are considered the preferred lab tests to use to help diagnose a heart attack, as they are indicators of cardiac muscle injury

or death. A series of blood tests for the enzymes performed over a 24-hour period are useful not only in confirming the diagnosis of heart attack, but the changes in their levels over time also correlate with the amount of heart muscle that has died.

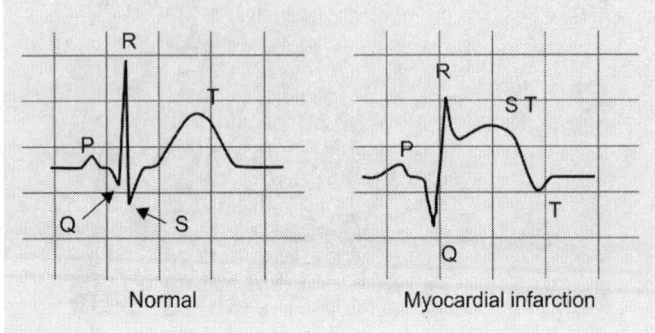

Fig. 3.10: ECG in myocardial infarction

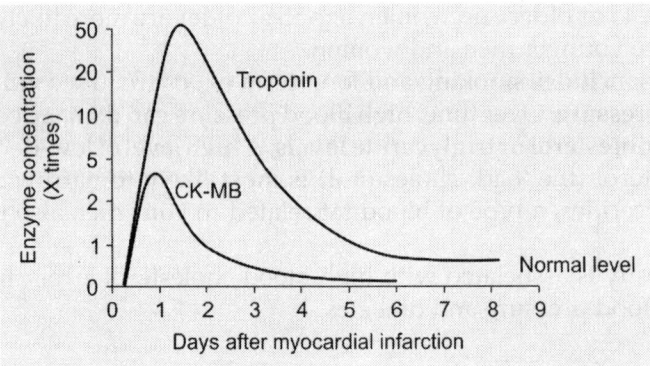

Fig. 3.11: Serum enzyme levels in myocardial infarction (CK-MB, creatine kinase MB)

Complications of MI

More important complications include:
- Cardiogenic shock
- Cardiac arrhythmias (ventricular tachycardia or ventricular fibrillation are life-threatening complications).
- Congestive heart failure

PATHOPHYSIOLOGIC BASIS OF TREATMENT

Treatment aims at immediate restoration of blood flow in the artery blocked by a blood clot followed by measures to prevent thrombosis again:
- Angioplasty and stent: Special tubing with an attached deflated balloon is threaded up to the coronary arteries. A stent is a wire mesh tube used to prop open an artery during angioplasty.
- Long-term antiplatelet therapy

<< **CONGESTIVE HEART FAILURE** >>

Congestive heart failure (CHF), or heart failure is defined as an inability of the heart to pump blood at a rate appropriate for the metabolic requirements of the tissues;

Aetiology: Important causes include:

➤ **Hypertension:** Due to high blood pressure, expulsion of blood requires more forceful ventricular contraction during each systole. Over time, the left ventricle initially undergoes hypertrophy and later it dilates leading to heart failure.

➤ **Coronary artery disease :** Myocardial infarction weakens the myocardium.

➤ **Valvular disease:** Disorders of aortic or mitral valve cause extra burden on the heart. Initially heart undergoes hypertrophy and later dilatation.

SYMPTOMS AND SIGNS

➤ Exercise intolerance
➤ Fatigue
➤ Dyspnoea on effort
➤ Cyanosis
➤ Ankle edema
➤ Distended neck veins
➤ Liver enlargement (hepatomegaly)
➤ Spleen enlargement (splenomegaly)
➤ Oedema feet (Fig. 3.12)
➤ Ascites (fluid in peritoneal cavity, abdomen) (Fig. 3.12)

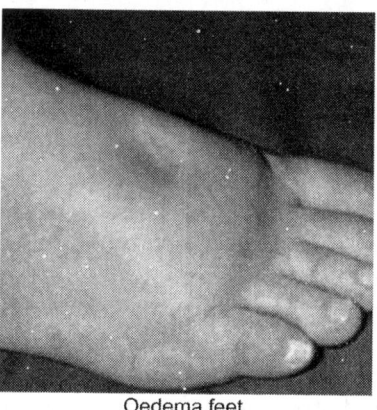 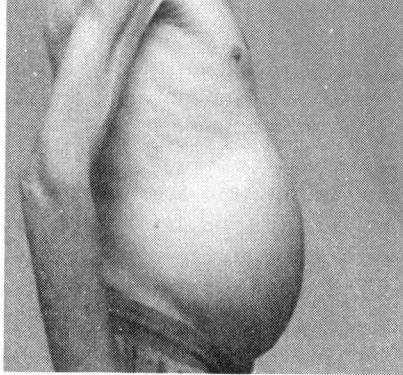

Oedema feet   Ascites

Fig. 3.12: Signs of right-sided heart failure

Pathophysiology of CHF

When the heart is unable to pump out sufficient amount of blood, a number of natural compensatory mechanisms are activated so as to improve the cardiac output and maintain normal perfusion of the vital organs. These mechanisms include:

➤ Frank-Starling mechanism
➤ Increased adrenergic discharge
➤ Regional redistribution of cardiac output
➤ Hormonal mechanisms

As you have learnt in physiology lectures, cardiac output can be increased by an increase in end-diastolic volume (EDV) (Starling mechanism) as well as an increase in sympathetic discharge to the heart. Both of these mechanisms are utilized to bring the failing heart to produce normal cardiac output. The other two compensatory mechanisms help in these primary mechanisms are:

1. **Frank-Starling mechanism:** As shown in Fig. 3.13, by working at greater EDV (Y in figure), the heart can pump out normal amount of blood. EDV is increased by the fourth compensatory mechanism mentioned above. (*See* (4) below).

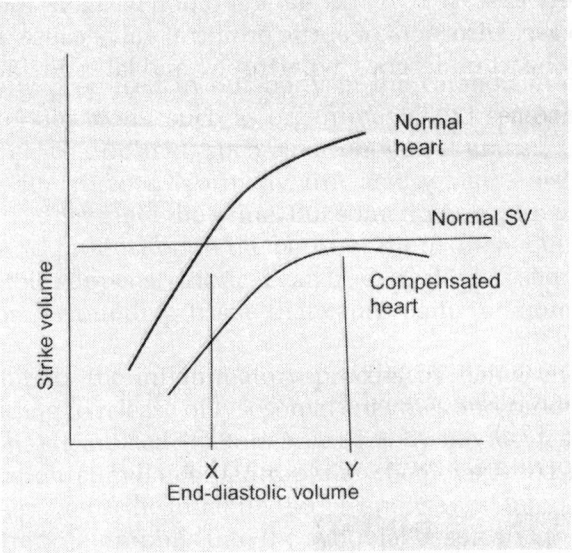

Fig. 3.13: Mechanism of compensation of a failing heart by Frank-Starling mechanism. Failing heart can improve stroke volume to normal by working at greater end-diastolic volume ("Y") instead of normal ("X"). (SV = stroke volume).

2. **Increased adrenergic discharge:** In the failing heart, depressed cardiac output is sensed by high pressure baroreceptors located in the carotid sinus and aortic arch, leading to a reflex increase in adrenergic discharge to the heart and blood vessels. In the heart, increased adrenergic discharge improves the cardiac output by increasing the heart rate as well as stroke volume (Fig. 3.14). In the blood vessels, it causes redistribution of cardiac output described next.

3. **Redistribution of cardiac output:** The redistribution of cardiac output serves as an important compensatory mechanism when cardiac output is reduced. Blood flow is redistributed so that the delivery of oxygen to vital organs, such as the brain and myocardium, is maintained at normal or near-normal levels, while flow to less critical areas, such as the cutaneous and muscular beds and viscera, is reduced. Vasoconstriction mediated by the adrenergic nervous system is largely responsible for this redistribution.

4. **Hormonal mechanisms:** Decreased cardiac output activates renin-angiotensin II-mechanism. Angiotensin II produces arteriolar constriction and increases thirst (increased water intake). It also increases aldosterone secretion, thereby producing salt and water retention in the kidney. As a result of both these factors, blood volume and thereby EDV is increased.

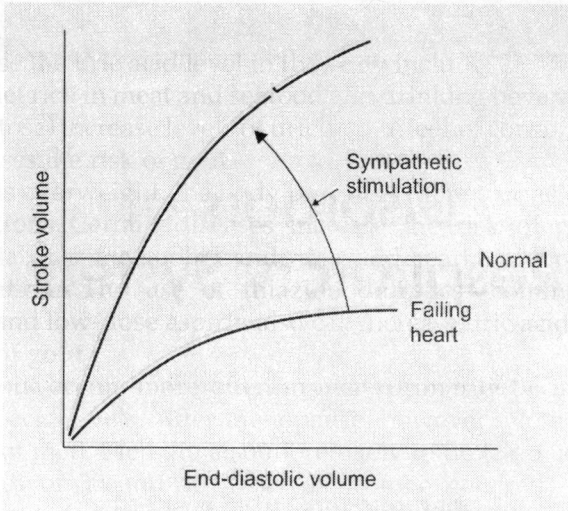

Fig. 3.14: Effect of increased sympathetic discharge on stroke volume in a failing heart

Decompensation

As the cardiac function gradually deteriorates, the compensatory mechanisms discussed above cannot maintain normal cardiac output. Moreover, excessive increase in EDV increases left and right atrial pressures resulting in congestion in the lungs and in systemic veins. At this point, congestive heart failure is said to have set in.

Pathophysiological Basis of Treatment

1. Strengthening the force of contraction of the heart: Digitalis.
2. Reducing salt and water retention: Diuretics
3. Reducing sympathetic over-activity: Beta blockers

Disorders of Respiratory System

Obstructive lung diseases are the second (after cardiovascular diseases) leading cause of death in the adult population in India. Obstructive lung disease refers to a group of diseases that share a common feature—*difficulty in expelling air from the lungs*.

➤ Asthma
➤ Chronic bronchitis
➤ Emphysema

All the three disorders have an increased airway resistance, but, caused by a different mechanism in each case. However, often there is an overlap (Fig. 4.1). In old cases of bronchial asthma, some element of emphysema develops. In chronic bronchitis, some element of bronchospasm is commonly present. Chronic bronchitis and emphysema are considered a spectrum of a chronic obstructive pulmonary disease (COPD) with some patients showing dominantly bronchitis, while others show dominantly emphysema.

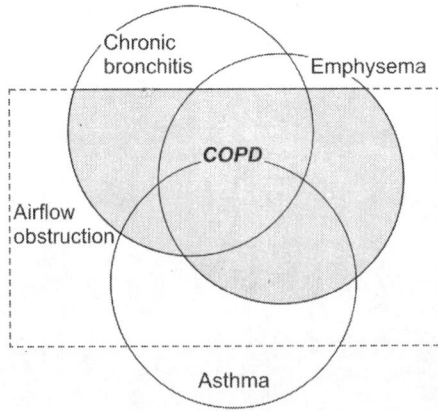

Fig. 4.1: Airway obstruction is a feature common to bronchial asthma, chronic bronchitis and emphysema.

In bronchial asthma, chronic bronchitis and emphysema, the common factor is increased airway resistance. *Pathogenesis and pathophysiology of obstructive lung disease can be explained only if the reader is familiar with the role of mucociliary clearance in respiratory mucosa and physiology of airway resistance.*

Mucociliary Clearance

From trachea down to the terminal bronchioles, the respiratory mucosa is characterized by the presence of cilia, goblet cells, and submucosal mucous glands. The cilia are covered with a blanket of mucus, which traps any incoming particle greater than 5 μ size. The ciliary movement of adjacent cells is so coordinated that it produces waves of ciliary motions from distal to the proximal parts of tracheo-bronchial tree (Fig. 4.2). As a result, mucus blanket on the top of cilia laden with dust particles or bacteria is propelled upwards till it reaches the oropharynx, where it is swallowed or expectorated. Mucociliary clearance is a critical factor in the protection of upper respiratory tract.

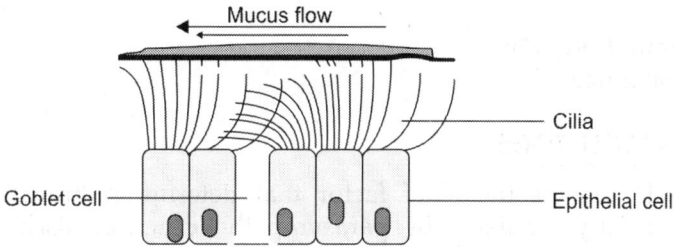

Fig. 4.2: Mucociliary clearance

AIRWAY RESISTANCE

Resistance in the airways (R_{aw}) is basically determined by same factors that determine vascular resistance:

$$R_{aw} = \frac{8nL}{\pi r4}$$

n = gas viscosity; L = airway length; r = radius

In the airways, the variable factor is radius of the airways. A given reduction in the radius of bronchi results in fourfold increase in airway resistance. Even 4% reduction in airway diameter doubles the airway resistance (Fig. 4.3).

LOWER AIRWAY RESISTANCE

The physiological control of airway resistance lies in the medium-sized bronchi (2–4 mm diameter). These airways contain, besides supporting cartilage, large amount of smooth muscle. Smooth muscle contraction can substantially increase airway resistance by reducing airway radius. The lumen of these bronchi can be altered by the following factors:

➢ Bronchomotor muscle tone
➢ Radial traction by lung parenchyma

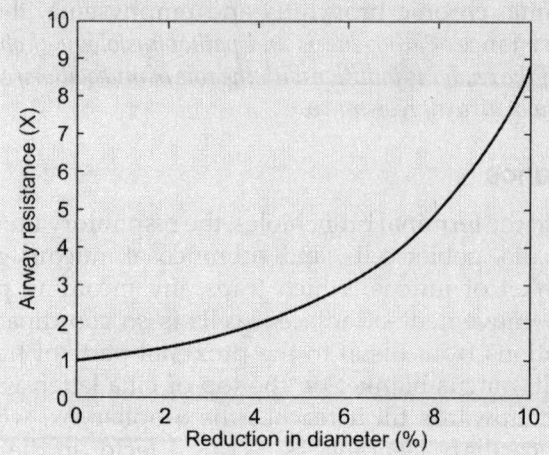

Fig. 4.3: Effect of reduction in airway diameter on airway resistance

➤ Transmural pressure
➤ Luminal mucus

BRONCHIAL MUSCLE TONE

Bronchial muscle tone is the chief factor that determines bronchial lumen size (Fig. 4.4). It is chiefly regulated by parasympathetic neural discharge. In allergic asthma, a large number of local chemical mediators, such as histamine, prostaglandins, leukotrienes, kinins, etc. are released. All these mediators produce varying degree of bronchial muscle spasm. In chronic bronchitis also, there is some degree of bronchospasm. Circulating epinephrine can produce bronchodilation by acting on β_2 receptors present on the bronchial smooth muscle. β_2 agonists are used in the treatment of bronchial asthma.

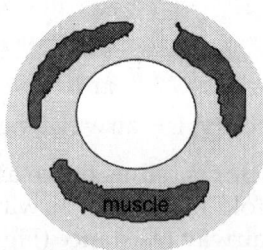

Fig. 4.4: Smooth muscle in a bronchiole

Radial Traction by Lung Parenchyma

Bronchi and bronchioles are surrounded by lung parenchyma, whose constant pull helps the patency of the airways. This supportive action is called radial traction. Parenchymal destructive diseases, such as emphysema, cause loss of radial traction. As a result, small airways collapse (Fig. 4.5). That is the chief mechanism of bronchial narrowing in emphysema.

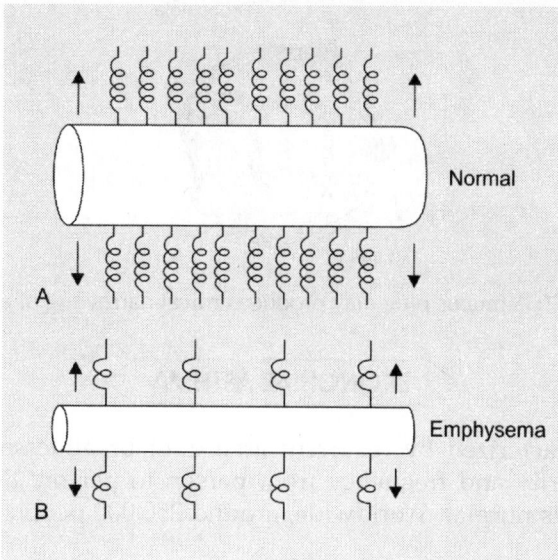

Fig. 4.5: Effect of loss of radial traction on bronchiolar lumen in an emphysema

Transmural Pressure

During inspiration, intrapleural pressure is negative with respect to intrapulmonary pressure which helps to keep airways open. Similar situation exists during tidal expiration also. However, during forced expiration, intrapleural pressure becomes strongly positive, which tends to cause dynamic airway collapse (Fig. 4.6). In emphysema, as explained later, expiration is brought about by active contraction of expiratory muscles. The dynamic airway collapse causes expiratory flow limitations, i.e. beyond a point, increased expiratory effort does not produce further increase in air outflow. The problem is worsened in emphysema due to loss of radial traction, as well.

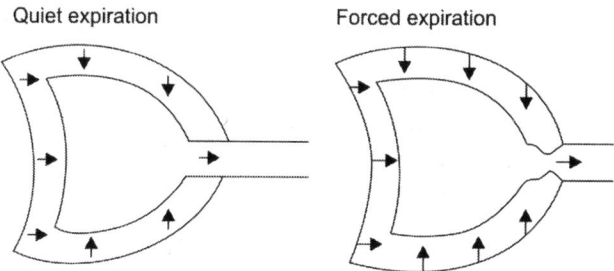

Fig. 4.6: Effect of positive transmural pressure on airway lumen (dynamic collapse of bronchiole in lower picture)

Mucus in Airways

The presence of mucus or other extraneous material in the airway lumen increases airway resistance (Fig. 4.7). Cigarette smoking or respiratory infections enhance the secretion of submucosal mucous glands as well as mucosal goblet cells in the respiratory tract.

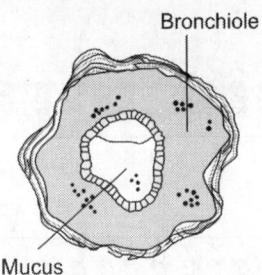

Fig. 4.7: A mucus plug may produce critical narrowing of airway

BRONCHIAL ASTHMA

It is a disease characterized by recurrent attacks of breathlessness and wheezing, which vary in severity and frequency from person to person. Between the attacks, patient's breathing is normal. Worldwide, around 250,000 people die every year as a result of asthma.

Symptoms

➢ Wheezing (a whistling sound arising from the lung during breathing)
➢ Tightness in the chest
➢ Shortness of breath
➢ Trouble sleeping caused by shortness of breath, coughing or wheezing
➢ Coughing or wheezing attacks that are worsened by a respiratory virus, such as a cold or the flu

Asthma Triggers

Exposure to various irritants and substances that trigger allergies (allergens) can trigger signs and symptoms of asthma. Asthma triggers are different from person to person and can include:

➢ Airborne substances, such as pollen, dust mites, mold spores, pet dander or particles of cockroach waste
➢ Respiratory infections, such as the common cold
➢ Physical activity (exercise-induced asthma)
➢ Cold air
➢ Air pollutants and irritants, such as smoke

PATHOGENESIS

The pathology of bronchial asthma consists of reversible bronchial narrowing associated with spasm of smooth muscle in the wall of airways (bronchi). The airway hyper-responsiveness is the fundamental disorder. The airway smooth muscle shows an exaggerated response to a variety of triggers such as seasonal outdoor allergens (pollens) or allergens derived from house dust, mites present in carpets, beds or domestic animals or cockroaches.

There is a genetic predisposition to bronchial asthma. A substantial percentage of asthmatic patients have elevated IgE levels (a sign of allergic predisposition) and history of additional allergic disorders.

Histological examination of small bronchi reveals epithelial damage, hypertrophy and hyperplasia of bronchial smooth muscle, enlargement of mucous glands, increased number of goblet cells and infiltration of bronchial wall with eosinophils and lymphocytes (Fig. 4.8). The inflamed tissues respond to any of the triggers by release of mediators such as histamine and bradykinin by the mast cells and eosinophils in the bronchial mucosa. These mediators produce bronchospasm and increased mucus secretion. The combined effect of bronchoconstriction and increased mucus secretion produces a critical narrowing of airways and increased airway resistance, especially during expiratory phase. During asthmatic attack, though breathing difficulty is felt during inspiratory phases, it becomes worse during expiratory phases of respiratory cycles.

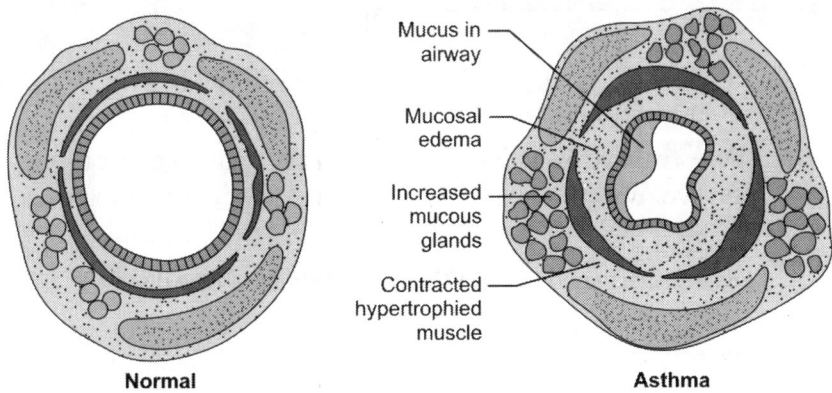

Normal   Asthma

Fig. 4.8: Histological changes in the bronchiole in bronchial asthma

Confirmatory Pulmonary Function Tests

➤ Forced vital capacity (FVC) is decreased
➤ Forced expiratory volume 1st second/vital capacity ratio (FEV_1/FVC ratio) is decreased (Fig. 4.9).
➤ Peak expiratory flow rate (PEFR) decreased.
➤ Increase in FEV_1/ VC ratio and PEFR when tested after inhalation of a bronchodilator drug (Fig. 4.10).

Risk Factors

➤ Family history.
➤ Viral respiratory infections during infancy and childhood.
➤ Other allergies: Having an allergic condition, such as eczema or allergic rhinitis is a risk factor for developing asthma.
➤ Smoking.
➤ Air pollution.
➤ Obesity.

Complications

➤ Frequent attacks of bronchial asthma interfere with day-to-day life.
➤ Acute severe asthma may progress to a life-threatening condition known as status asthmaticus.
➤ COPD (emphysema) in later life.

Pathophysiological basis of treatment: An attack of bronchial asthma can be terminated by administration of a bronchodilator drug.

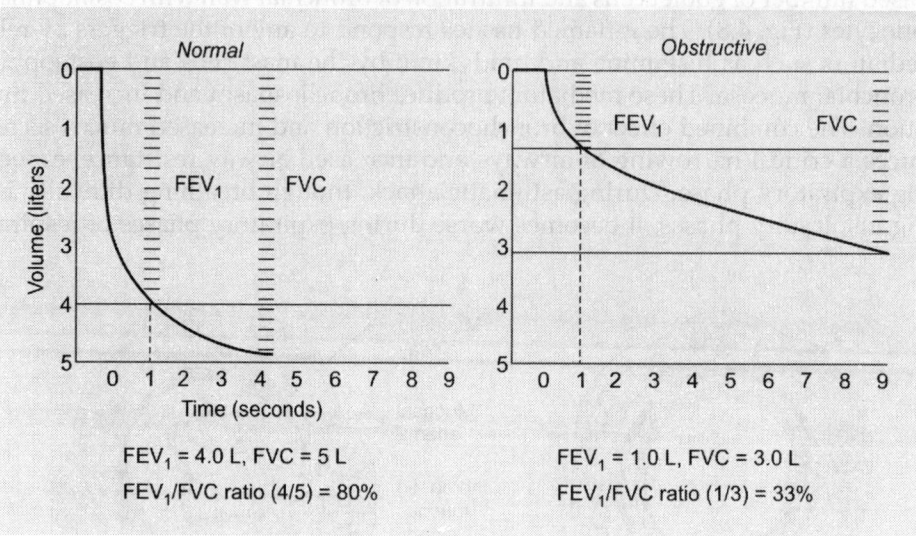

$FEV_1 = 4.0\ L,\ FVC = 5\ L$
FEV_1/FVC ratio $(4/5) = 80\%$

$FEV_1 = 1.0\ L,\ FVC = 3.0\ L$
FEV_1/FVC ratio $(1/3) = 33\%$

Fig. 4.9: Decreased FEV_1/ FVC ratio in obstructive lung disease

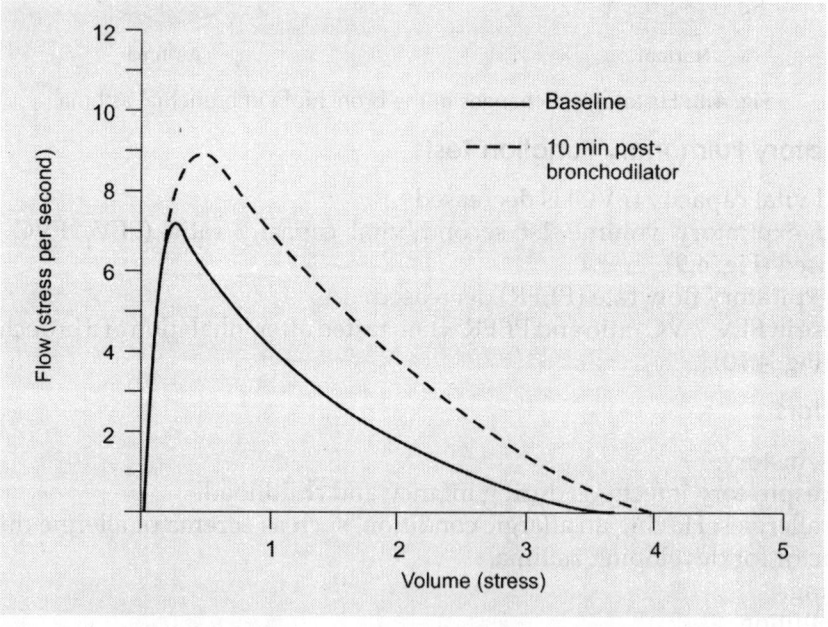

Fig. 4.10: Increased flow rate after administration of a bronchodilator in a case of bronchial asthma

CHRONIC OBSTRUCTIVE PULMONARY DISEASE (COPD)

COPD is defined as a chronic, slowly progressive disorder characterized by airflow obstruction *which continues over several months*. Bronchial asthma, though involves airflow obstruction, is excluded by this definition. The COPD starts as chronic bronchitis, which over the years develops into emphysema.

SYMPTOMS AND SIGNS

Signs and symptoms of COPD may include:
➢ Cough and copious sputum
➢ Shortness of breath, especially during physical activities
➢ Wheezing
➢ Chest tightness
➢ Blueness of the lips or fingernail beds (cyanosis) (later stages)
➢ Frequent respiratory infections
➢ Swelling in ankles, feet (later stages)

AETIOLOGY

1. **Cigarette smoking:** Cigarette smoking is considered to be the most important cause of COPD. Cigarette smoke contributes to the development of COPD through a number of mechanisms:
   ➢ Inhibits ciliary clearance function in bronchial mucosa
   ➢ Inhibits function of alveolar macrophages
   ➢ Causes hypertrophy of goblet cells and mucous glands
   ➢ Provokes release of elastase from polymorphonuclear neutrophils
   ➢ Causes destruction of alveolar parenchyma by inhibiting α_1-antitrypsin
   ➢ Increases airway resistance by stimulating irritant receptors
2. **Air pollutants:** Almost 3 billion people worldwide use biomass and coal as their main source of energy for cooking, heating, and other household needs. In these communities, indoor air pollution is responsible for a greater fraction of COPD risk than smoking or outdoor air pollution. Biomass fuels used by women for cooking account for the high prevalence of COPD among nonsmoking women in parts of the Middle East, Africa and Asia. Indoor air pollution resulting from the burning of wood and other biomass fuels is estimated to kill two million women and children each year.
3. Frequent lower respiratory infections during childhood.
4. Congenital alpha-1 antitrypsin deficiency.
5. Occupational dusts and chemicals (such as vapours, irritants, and fumes)

PATHOPHYSIOLOGY

COPD with Predominant Bronchitis

In such patients, the major pathology is increased activity of hypertrophic and hyperplastic mucus secreting apparatus (goblet cells and mucous glands) throughout large and small airways (Fig. 4.11). Excessive production of thick and viscid mucus results in characteristic cough and copious purulent sputum. The airway obstruction is primarily due to these changes in the terminal bronchioles. Besides intraluminal secretions, some degree of bronchospasm, or thickening of airway wall by edema, inflammation or fibrosis contribute to the increased airway resistance. A component of airway hyper-responsiveness may further aggravate bronchial obstruction resulting in what is called asthmatic bronchitis.

In relatively "pure" chronic bronchitis, pulmonary parenchyma is mostly intact and oxygen diffusion capacity is near normal. However, the patient shows more marked decrease in arterial pO_2 (45–50 mmHg) as well as moderately elevated pCO_2

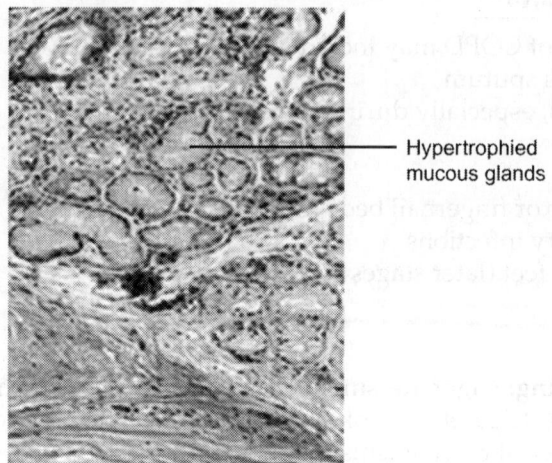

Hypertrophied mucous glands

Fig. 4.11: Histological picture of a bronchus in chronic bronchitis

(50–60 mmHg) and marked polycythaemia. The abnormalities in blood gases arise chiefly from uneven ventilation/perfusion in different parts of the lungs. Some bronchioles are obstructed by mucus/inflammation/edema causing marked decrease in ventilation, but fairly well-maintained perfusion. The physiological shunts lead to hypoxia and polycythaemia.

Increased pulmonary vascular resistance is important feature of chronic bronchitis. It mainly results from chronic hypoxia. Other contributory factors include increased polycythaemia, increased pCO_2 and acidosis.

Confirmatory Pulmonary Function Tests

➢ Forced vital capacity (FVC) is decreased
➢ Forced expiratory volume 1st second/vital capacity ratio (FEV_1/FVC ratio) is decreased.
➢ Peak expiratory flow rate (PEFR) decreased.
➢ There is no significant improvement in FEV_1/FVC ratio and PEFR when tested after inhalation of a bronchodilator drug.
➢ Total lung capacity (TLC) is normal.

COPD with Prominent Emphysema

In such a patient, the primary problem is degeneration of alveolar tissue. The destruction of air space walls reduces the surface area available for the exchange of oxygen and carbon dioxide during breathing. It also reduces the elasticity of the lung itself, which results in a loss of support for the airways that are embedded in the lung (Figs 4.5 and 4.12), leading to a *decrease in elastic recoil of the lungs*. Therefore, the force that normally drives air out of lungs during expiration decreases. Due to disruption of the alveolar septa, the support that keeps the small airways open due to transmural pressure is lost.

Due to loss of elastic fibers, compliance of the lungs increases, the lungs are inflated to a larger volume for a given degree of increase in intrapulmonary pressure. The total lung capacity increases and lungs remain permanently inflated. Residual volume and functional residual capacity are both increased. The chest becomes barrel-shaped. The diaphragm remains permanently flattened (Fig. 4.13). As a result, diaphragm contraction cannot contribute to inspiratory effort. Inspiration is produced by the contraction of external intercostals only. Due to loss of elastic fibers, expiration is produced by active contraction of expiratory muscles rather than by passive recoil of elastic fibers. This results in dyspnoea and increased energy cost of work of breathing.

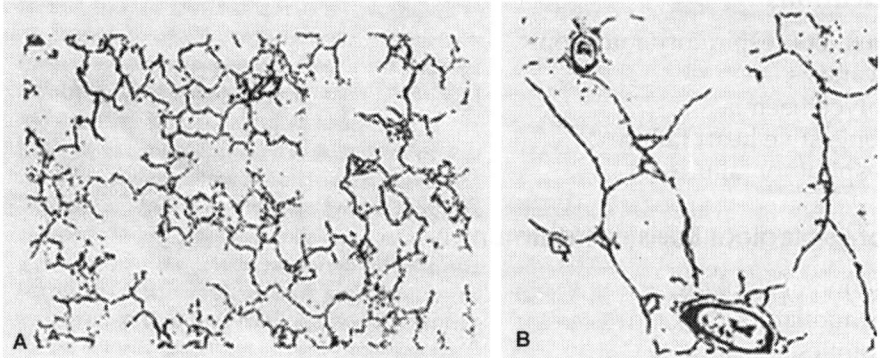

Fig. 4.12: Microscopic appearance of lungs in emphysema (B) as compared to normal (A)

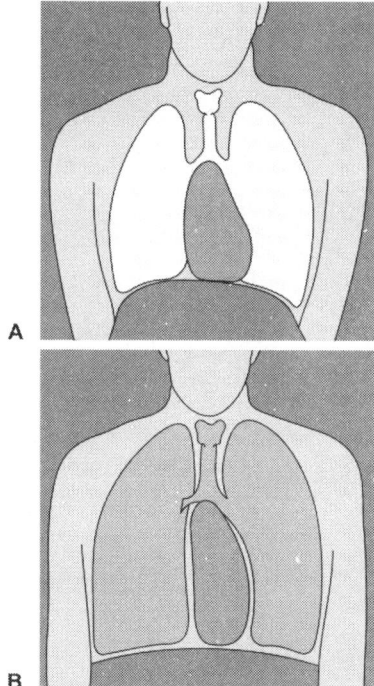

Fig. 4.13: Effect of hyperinflation of lungs in emphysema on the position of diaphragm during expiration (B). Compare with normal (A)

Confirmatory Pulmonary Function Tests

➤ Forced vital capacity (FVC) is decreased
➤ Forced expiratory volume 1st second/vital capacity ratio (FEV_1/FVC ratio) is decreased.
➤ Peak expiratory flow rate (PEFR) decreased.
➤ There is no significant improvement in FEV_1/FVC ratio and PEFR when tested after inhalation of a bronchodilator drug.
➤ Total lung capacity (TLC) is increased.

Complications

1. Frequent respiratory infections
2. Cyanosis
3. Polycythaemia
4. Congestive heart failure
5. Respiratory failure

Pathophysiological Basis of Treatment

➤ Cessation of smoking
➤ Bronchodilators
➤ Antibiotics
➤ Oxygen therapy when the patient has cyanosis in later stages of COPD
➤ Treatment of congestive heart failure (in later stages)

Disorders of Renal System

Kidney failure is defined as a condition when the kidneys are no longer able to remove the waste products from the body leading to their accumulation in the blood. This can cause unsafe levels of waste products to build up. This is known as kidney (or renal) failure. Unless it is treated, this can cause death. There are 2 main types of kidney (renal) failure: **Acute** (sudden) and **chronic** (over time).

ACUTE RENAL FAILURE (ARF)

Acute renal failure is traditionally defined as an abrupt (within 48 hours) reduction in the rate of glomerular filtration, which manifests clinically as an abrupt and sustained increase in the serum levels of urea and creatinine with an associated disruption of salt and water homeostasis. The elevation of blood urea nitrogen (BUN) and serum creatinine levels is known as **azotaemia.** Azotaemia is biochemical evidence of renal failure. (The normal range for blood urea is 20–40 mg/dl and the normal range for serum creatinine is 0.7–1.4 mg/dl.)

SYMPTOMS OF ACUTE RENAL FAILURE (ARF)

➢ Decrease in urine output (oliguria)
➢ Swelling of the hands, feet and face (edema)
➢ Fatigue
➢ Nausea
➢ Confusion
➢ Seizures
➢ Coma
➢ Abnormal blood and urine tests
➢ High blood pressure

PATHOGENESIS OF ARF

Acute renal failure is classified as (Fig. 5.1):

1. **Pre-renal azotaemia:** It typically results from a severe decrease in renal blood flow due to severe blood loss leading to hypotension or severe dehydration. In

this type of ARF, nephrons are normal. If blood volume is restored to normal, patient makes quick recovery.

2. **Renal azotaemia:** It occurs in response to cytotoxic, ischemic, or inflammatory insults to the kidney, with structural and functional damage to the nephrons. It is the most serious type of ARF. Recovery is slow.

3. **Post-renal azotaemia:** It includes disorders associated with obstruction of the urinary tract, e.g. obstruction to urethra by enlarged prostate gland in the males. Recovery is rapid after removal of the obstruction.

With proper and timely treatment, most forms of ARI are reversible, since kidney is a unique organ which can recover completely even after almost complete loss of renal function.

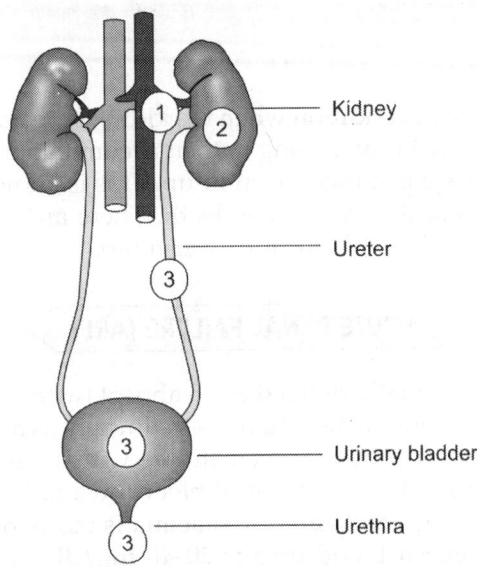

Fig. 5.1: Acute renal failure. (1) Pre-renal azotaemia; (2) renal azotaemia; (3) post-renal azotaemia

Prerenal Azotaemia

Causes

➤ **Hypovolemia:** Hemorrhage, burns, dehydration, diuretics.
➤ **Low cardiac output:** Myocardial infarction, pulmonary embolism, CHF.
➤ **Shock:** Sepsis, anaphylaxis.

Prerenal azotaemia represents the most common form (50 to 80%) of acute kidney failure and often leads to *renal azotaemia*, if it is not promptly corrected. All the conditions mentioned above cause renal hypoperfusion due to a decrease in the circulatory blood volume. A decrease in circulating blood volume activates high pressure arterial baroreceptors leading to a reflex increase in sympathetic discharge, severe renal vasoconstriction and a tendency to reduced GFR. When the renal hypoperfusion is severe, the renal compensatory mechanisms fail, resulting in a severe reduction in GFR and azotaemia results. Blood levels of urea or creatinine begin to rise only when GFR falls to less than 50% of normal (Fig. 5.2). Any further delay in treatment of hypovolemia results in such an intense renal vasoconstriction that the renal tubular epithelium undergoes ischemic necrosis (*acute tubular necrosis, ATN*).

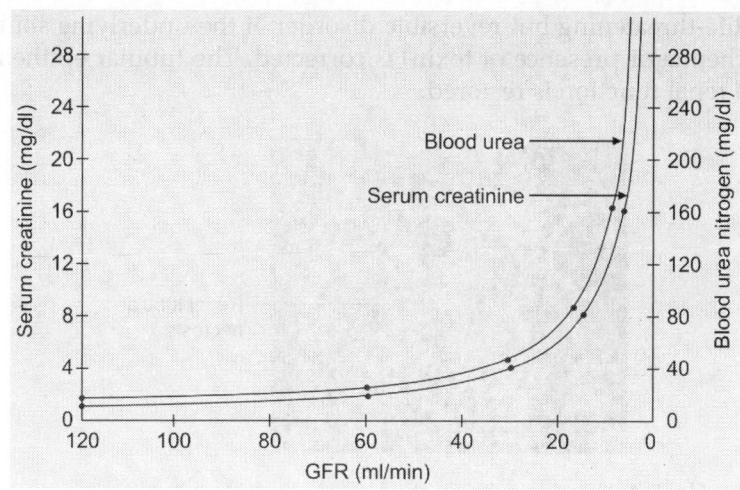

Fig. 5.2: Relation between GFR and serum creatinine or blood urea levels

Renal Azotaemia

One specific clinical disorder called the *acute tubular necrosis (ATN)* accounts for most of the cases of intrinsic azotaemia. It is produced by injury to renal parenchyma.

Pathogenesis of Acute Tubular Necrosis

Acute tubular necrosis (ATN) is the term used to designate acute kidney injury resulting from damage to the tubules. The major causes of ATN are:
1. **Ischaemic:** Resulting from severe or protracted decrease in renal perfusion (complication of prerenal azotaemia).
2. **Nephrotoxicity:** Resulting from a variety of exogenous drugs that damage the kidneys.
3. **Hemoglobinuria:** In case of incompatible blood transfusion, there is severe intravascular haemolysis leading to haemoglobinuria. Presence of haemoglobin in the kidney damages the renal tubules.

Pathology

Regardless of the pathogenesis, ATN is characterized by a common set of morphological changes. These morphologic changes usually appear in a segmental pattern with some segments of the nephron, such as the proximal tubule and thick ascending loop of Henle which are more susceptible than others parts of nephron (Fig. 5.3).

Tubular Epithelium

The tubular epithelium undergoes necrosis which can be seen by denudation of tubular epithelial cells. In some cases the tubular basement membrane may rupture.

Tubular Lumen

The denuded and necrotic tubular epithelial cells ultimately fall into the tubular lumen and often plug the tubule in the form of proteinaceous casts. When ATN is initiated by haemolysis, heme pigment may be precipitated in the luminal debris.

ATN is a life-threatening but reversible disorder, if the underlying source of injury (i.e. renal ischemia or presence of toxin) is corrected. The tubular epithelium rapidly recovers and renal function is restored.

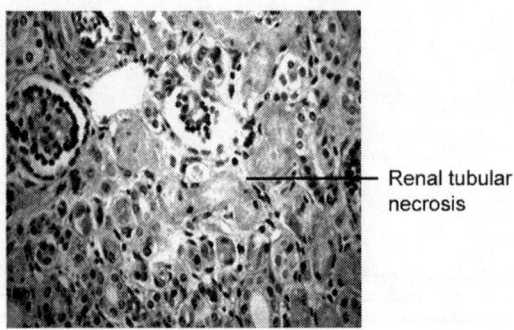

Renal tubular necrosis

Fig. 5.3: Histological picture of kidney in acute tubular necrosis

Post-renal Azotaemia

Approximately 5–10% cases of acute azotaemia are due to obstruction to the urinary tract. Since normal kidney function can be achieved by a single kidney, post-renal azotaemia can occur if there is:

➤ Obstruction of bladder neck (prostate pathology) or urethra.

➤ Bilateral ureteric obstruction, or

➤ Unilateral ureteric obstruction in a patient with only one functioning kidney.

Prostatic disease is the most common cause of post-renal azotaemia. Continued formation of urine against the backdrop of obstruction to outflow causes an increase in intraluminal pressure upstream the site of obstruction. Thus, there is a gradual distension ureters, renal pelvis and calyces (hydronephrosis). Ultimately, when the intraluminal pressure in the Bowman's capsule becomes equal to hydrostatic pressure in the glomerular capillaries, filtration ceases. Cessation in glomerular filtration leads to azotaemia, acidosis, fluid overload, and hyperkalaemia. *Post-renal azotaemia is the most common cause of complete anuria, because the basic cause is mechanical.* In pre-renal and renal types of ARI, complete renal shutdown seldom occurs.

With relief of obstruction within 48 hours of onset, there is evidence that relatively complete recovery of GFR can be achieved within a week. Prolonged obstruction can lead to tubular atrophy and irreversible renal fibrosis.

CHRONIC RENAL FAILURE

Chronic renal failure (CRF) refers to a decline in the glomerular filtration rate caused by a variety of diseases, such as diabetes, glomerulonephritis, and polycystic kidney disease. Patients with CRF have a high prevalence of hypertension. Whether hypertension is a cause or a result of CRF remains debatable. Chronic renal failure is a continuous process that begins when some nephrons begin to be lost and ends when the remnant nephrons can sustain life no longer.

Classification: Staging of chronic kidney disease is a way of quantifying the severity of CKD. Chronic kidney disease has been classified into 5 stages (Table 5.1). The end-stage, when symptoms begin to appear, is known as **uremia**

Table 5.1	Stages of chronic kidney disease	
Stage	*Description*	*Glomerular filtration rate (ml/min)*
At increased risk	**Risk factors** for kidney disease (e.g. diabetes, high blood pressure, family history, older age, ethnic group)	More than 90
1.	Kidney damage (protein in the urine) and **normal** GFR	More than 90
2.	Kidney damage and **mild** decrease in GFR	60 to 89
3.	**Moderate** decrease in GFR	30 to 59
4.	**Severe** decrease in GFR	15 to 29
5.	**Kidney failure** (dialysis or kidney transplant needed)	Less than 15

RISK FACTORS

Factors that may increase risk of chronic kidney disease include:
➤ Diabetes
➤ High blood pressure
➤ cardiovascular disease
➤ Smoking
➤ Obesity
➤ Family history of kidney disease
➤ Abnormal kidney structure
➤ Older age

Symptoms

➤ Nausea
➤ Vomiting
➤ Loss of appetite
➤ Fatigue and weakness
➤ Decreased mental sharpness
➤ Muscle twitches and cramps
➤ Swelling of feet and ankles
➤ Persistent itching
➤ Shortness of breath
➤ High blood pressure that is difficult to control

Aetiology

➤ Diabetes
➤ High blood pressure
➤ Glomerulonephritis, an inflammation of the kidney's glomeruli
➤ Polycystic kidney disease
➤ Prolonged obstruction of the urinary tract, from conditions such as enlarged prostate, kidney stones and some cancers
➤ Recurrent kidney infection, also called pyelonephritis

Pathology

The microscopic appearance of the "end stage kidney" is similar regardless of cause, which is why a biopsy in a patient with chronic renal failure yields little useful information. The **cortex** is fibrotic, the **glomeruli** are sclerotic, there are scattered chronic inflammatory cell infiltrates, and the **arteries** are thickened. Tubules are often dilated and filled with pink casts (Fig. 5.4).

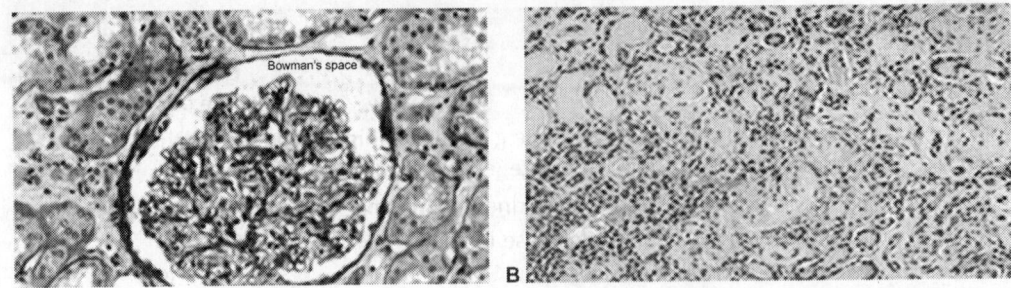

Fig. 5.4: Kidney, normal (A) and in end-stage kidney disease (B)

PATHOPHYSIOLOGY OF UREMIA (END-STAGE RENAL FAILURE)

The most characteristic features of uremia are:

1. Accumulation of nitrogenous waste products (urea, creatinine, uric acid, etc.) in the blood.
2. Metabolic acidosis (due to failure of H^+ excretion).
3. Hyperkalaemia (due to failure of K^+ excretion).
4. Anemia (deficiency of erythropoietin).
5. Uremic coma

The multiple organ failure in a uremic patient is due to the accumulation of some toxin(s) in the blood. However, the exact nature of the toxin(s) has not yet been identified. The final end product of carbohydrate and fat metabolisms is CO_2 (and water), which can be easily excreted by the lungs. The products of protein metabolism consist of a number of nitrogenous waste products which can be excreted only by the kidneys. Their accumulation in the blood consequent to renal failure is believed to be the cause of uremic toxicity.

1. **General cellular dysfunction:** The most basic abnormality in uremia, at cellular level, is partial inhibition of Na^+-K^+ pump, leading to a reduction in transmembrane potential, an increase in intracellular Na^+ and a decrease in intracellular K^+ concentrations. The most prominent result is an osmotically-induced overhydration of the cells. That is why salt and water retention is one of the important features of uremic syndrome. Overhydration of cerebral neurons is believed to be one of the factors contributing to the development of uremic encephalopathy. Additional factors decreasing *intracellular* K^+ concentration include metabolic acidosis, poor dietary intake of K^+, excessive losses due to vomiting, diarrhoea or diuretics.

2. **Hypothermia:** The sodium–potassium pump is the major consumer of ATP and hence the major cause of thermogenesis. Therefore, uremic patients have reduced energy metabolism, reduced BMR, subnormal body temperature and increased tendency to develop hypothermia.

3. **Anemia and immune dysfunction:** Anemia is a regular feature of uremia. Normochromic normocytic anemia principally develops from decreased renal synthesis of erythropoietin, the hormone responsible for bone marrow stimulation for red blood cell production. Anemia associated with renal failure can be observed when the glomerular filtration rate (GFR) is less than 50 ml/min or when the serum creatinine is greater than 2 mg/dl. In the course of the disease,

it becomes more severe as the GFR progressively decreases with the availability of less viable renal mass.

Atrophy of lymphoid tissue leading to lymphopaenia is common. Neutrophil count is usually normal. Uremic patients have impaired acute inflammatory response because of functional defects in neutrophils, monocytes and lymphocytes. Therefore, uremic patients are more prone to infections. Clotting defects may also occur.

4. **Renal osteodystrophy:** In a uremic patient, a number of abnormalities of the calcium, phosphate and vitamin D metabolisms, such as hypocalcemia, hyperphosphatemia, increased PTH levels, and metabolic acidosis ultimately lead to renal bone disease (renal osteodystrophy). Renal osteodystrophy is characterized by areas of osteomalacia and osteoporosis, and even osteosclerosis in various bones. These changes are seen more often in children or adults with slowly progressive chronic renal failure.

5. **Acidosis:** Acidosis is another major metabolic abnormality associated with uremia. Metabolic acid–base regulation is controlled primarily by tubular cells of the kidney, while respiratory compensation is accomplished in the lungs. Failure to secrete hydrogen ions and impaired excretion of ammonium may initially contribute to metabolic acidosis. In uremia, metabolic acidosis may contribute to other clinical abnormalities, such as hyperventilation, anorexia, stupor, congestive heart failure, and muscle weakness. Uremic patients are likely to go into severe acidosis on exposure to exogenous acids, e.g. high protein diet or endogenous acids such as lactic acid.

6. **Hyperkalemia:** As renal function declines, the nephron is unable to excrete a normal potassium load, which can lead to hyperkalemia if dietary intake remains constant. In addition, other metabolic abnormalities, such as acidosis, may contribute to decreased potassium excretion and lead to hyperkalemia. The *extracellular K^+* concentration begins to rise progressively with the degree of azotaemia. Serum K^+ level of greater than 6.5 mEq/L is a clinical emergency.

7. **Cardiovascular dysfunction:** Left ventricular hypertrophy is a common disorder found in approximately 75% of patients of chronic renal failure who have not yet undergone dialysis. Left ventricular hypertrophy is associated with increased ventricular thickness, arterial stiffening, coronary atherosclerosis, and/or coronary artery calcification. Patients are at increased risk for cardiac arrhythmias due to underlying hyperkalemia and metabolic acidosis. Renal dysfunction may contribute to associated fluid retention, which may lead to uncontrolled hypertension and congestive heart failure.

8. **Fluid and electrolyte imbalance:** In most cases of CRF, both total body sodium and water are increased and therefore the expansion of ECF volume may not be apparent. However, the patient is intolerant to both excessive salt intake and salt depletion. Excessive salt intake aggravates hypertension, congestive heart failure, ascites or edema.

   Uremic patients also have impaired mechanisms for salt and water conservation. There are more prone to volume depletion in states of sodium losses (vomiting, diarrhoea, fever) which may lead to orthostatic hypotension or circulatory shock. Volume depletion may produce further deterioration of renal function.

9. **Uremic neuropathy:** Uremic neuropathy is a distal sensorimotor polyneuropathy caused by uraemic toxins. The severity of neuropathy is correlated strongly with

the severity of the renal insufficiency. Paresthesias are the most common and usually the earliest symptom. Increased pain sensation is a prominent symptom. Weakness of lower extremities and atrophy follow the sensory symptoms. As disease progresses, symptoms move proximally and involve the upper extremities. Muscle cramps and restless legs syndrome were reported by 67% of uremic patients. Patients report that crawling, prickling, and itching sensations in their lower extremities are relieved partially by movement of the affected limb.

10. **Uremic encephalopathy:** Uremic encephalopathy (UE) is one of many manifestations of renal failure. Its exact cause is unknown. Accumulating metabolites of proteins and amino acids affect the entire neuraxis. No single abnormality can be precisely correlated with the clinical features of UE. Early symptoms include an inability to concentrate, drowsiness and insomnia. Mild behavioral changes, loss of memory and errors of judgment soon follow. Flapping tremor, chorea, stupor, seizers and coma are seen in terminal stages.

11. **Malnutrition:** Malnutrition usually occurs as renal failure progresses and is manifested by anorexia, weight loss, loss of muscle mass, low cholesterol levels, low BUN levels in the setting of an elevated creatinine level and hypoalbuminemia. Co-morbid diseases, such as diabetes, congestive heart failure, or other diseases, that require reduced food intake or restrictions of certain foods may contribute to anorexia.

12. **Skin:** The classic skin finding in persons with uremia is *uraemic frost*, which is a fine residue, thought to consist of excreted urea left on the skin after evaporation of water. Patients may become hyperpigmented as uremia worsens. Uremic pruritus remains one of the most frustrating, common, and potentially disabling symptoms in patients with end-stage renal disease. The exact cause is not yet clear.

HEMODIALYSIS

Hemodialysis can be a life-saving measure in many types of *acute renal failure* produced by reversible pathological processes. Patients with chronic renal failure can also be kept alive for months or even years.

During hemodialysis, the patient's radial artery is connected to a long and coiled cellophane tube immersed in a dialysing fluid. The chemical composition of dialyzing fluid is similar to that of plasma except that it is free of the waste products, like urea, uric acid, etc. (Table 5.2).

Table 5.2 Composition of dialyzing fluid as compared to that of a typical uremic plasma		
	Uremic plasma	*Dialysate*
Electrolyte (mEq/L)		
Na^+	142	142
K^+	7	4
Ca^{++}	2	3
Mg^{++}	1.5	1.5
Cl^-	107	107
HCO_3^-	14	27
Lactate	1.2	1.2

Contd.

Table 5.2	Composition of dialyzing fluid as compared to that of a typical uremic plasma (Contd.)	
	Uremic plasma	**Dialysate**
HPO_4^{2-}	9	0
Urate	2	0
SO_4^{2-}	3	0
Non-electrolyte (mg%)		
Glucose	100	125
Urea	200	0
Creatinine	6	0

The patient's blood passes through the dialysing system and returns to a peripheral vein. The semipermeable cellophane membrane permits free diffusion of all the constituents of plasma except proteins. In this way, the dialysis of patient's blood removes the toxic waste products and restores normal electrolyte concentration in the plasma. The dialysing system is also known as the artificial kidney (Fig. 5.5).

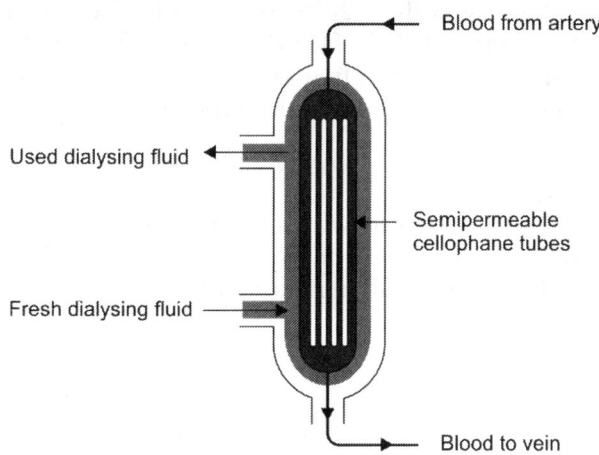

Fig. 5.5: Principle of hemodialysis

The hemodialysis is an expensive procedure and needs to be repeated almost every week. Therefore, it cannot be regarded as a remedy for irreversible renal failure caused by chronic renal diseases. With the recent advances in medical technology, such patients are treated by renal transplantation.

Haematological Disorders

◁ ANEMIA ▷

Anemia is a global health problem. About 25% of world population is anemic. Anemia is highly prevalent in India as well. In 2016, 51% of Indian women in the reproductive age group (15–49 years age) and 57% of children under the age of 5 years were found to be anemic. Surprisingly, 25% of Indian men were also found to be anemic. These statistics show that anemia is a national health problem in India.

DEFINITION

Anemia is defined as a condition in which the hemoglobin concentration is below the normal range, for the age and sex of the individual. In adults, the lower limit of the normal range is taken as 13 g/dL in males and 12 g/dL in females (or hematocrit below 40% in males and 35% in females).

SYMPTOMS

Subnormal levels of hemoglobin decrease the oxygen carrying capacity of the blood leading to deficiency of oxygen in the tissues (hypoxia). The function of tissues with high oxygen demand such as heart, brain and exercising muscles are most affected. The symptoms of anemia include
➢ Pale skin
➢ Tiredness
➢ Palpitation
➢ Easy fatigability
➢ Generalized muscle weakness
➢ Lethargy
➢ Headache
➢ Light-headedness
➢ Cold hands and feet
  The severity of these symptoms increases with the severity of anemia. WHO has classified anemia as mild, moderate and severe on the basis of hemoglobin concentration of the blood (Table 6.1).

Table 6.1	Classification of severity of anemia		
Anemia	**Hemoglobin concentration g/dL**		
	Mild	*Moderate*	*Severe*
Adult men	11.0–12.9	8.0–10.9	<8.0
Adult women	11.0–11.9	8.0–10.9	<8.0

When a patient is diagnosed as suffering from anemia, the treatment would depend on its aetiology (cause). However, before trying to find the cause, it is helpful to first classify anemia according to the red cell indices (laboratory classification) discussed below.

RED CELL INDICES

From the RBC count, hemoglobin concentration and hematocrit (PCV) value, certain indices (or absolute values) of the red cells of the person can be calculated. These absolute values are used in the *laboratory diagnosis of anemia*. The method of calculation and normal range of various red cell indices are shown in Table 6.2. On the basis of red cell indices, an anemia may be classified as (i) microcytic, normocytic or macrocytic, and (ii) hypochromic or normochromic. Once these indices are known, one can proceed to find out the cause.

Table 6.2	Calculation and normal range of red cell indices	
Absolute value	**Normal range**	**Calculation**
Mean corpuscular volume (MCV)	80–100 μ^3	$\dfrac{PCV\ (\%) \times 10}{RBC\ count\ (millions\ \mu^3)}$
Mean corpuscular hemoglobin (MCH)	26–34 pg	$\dfrac{Hb\ (g/dL) \times 10}{RBC\ count\ (millions\ \mu^3)}$
Mean corpuscular hemoglobin concentration (%)	32–38%	$\dfrac{Hb\ (g/dL) \times 100}{PCV\ (\%)}$

AETIOLOGICAL CLASSIFICATION OF ANEMIAS

➢ Deficiency anemia
➢ Hemorrhagic anemia
➢ Haemolytic anemia
➢ Aplastic anemia

PATHOGENESIS OF ANEMIA

1. Deficiency Anemia

(a) Iron deficiency anemia

Iron deficiency is the commonest cause of anemia in the world. Iron deficiency results in deficient production of hemoglobin and the number of red blood cells. As explained below, it is more common in the females than in males. It is important economically because it diminishes the capability of individuals who are affected to perform physical labour, and it diminishes both growth and learning in children. Anemic patients seem to be more prone to infections.

Iron deficiency anemia is usually the end result of a long period of negative iron balance (iron intake is less than iron excretion). The daily requirement of iron in males is very little. Except malnourished individuals, males are not prone to develop iron deficiency anemia. Therefore, in a male patient with such type of anemia, causes such as gastrointestinal blood loss, malabsorption or hookworm infestation should be looked for.

Females in the reproductive age group are prone to develop iron deficiency because of loss of iron in menstruation, pregnancy and lactation. Excessive menstrual losses or repeated pregnancies are the usual causes of iron deficiency anemia in women. Gastric surgery and achlorhydria are other causes of iron deficiency anemia which may occur both in males and females.

Iron deficiency results in the production of a smaller number of red cells, which are not only deficient in haemoglobin (hypochromic), but also smaller in size (microcytic) (Fig. 6.1). Thus, in iron deficiency, the MCH is below 26 pg, MCHC below 32% and MCV below 80 μ^3. Severe iron deficiency not only interferes with erythropoiesis but also with cell division in many other tissues. Severe iron deficiency is associated with not only severe anemia, but also with disorders of tongue (atrophic glossitis), oesophagus (dysphagia) and nails (koilonychias, spoon-like nails). Iron deficiency can be easily treated by oral administration of Fe^{2+} salts.

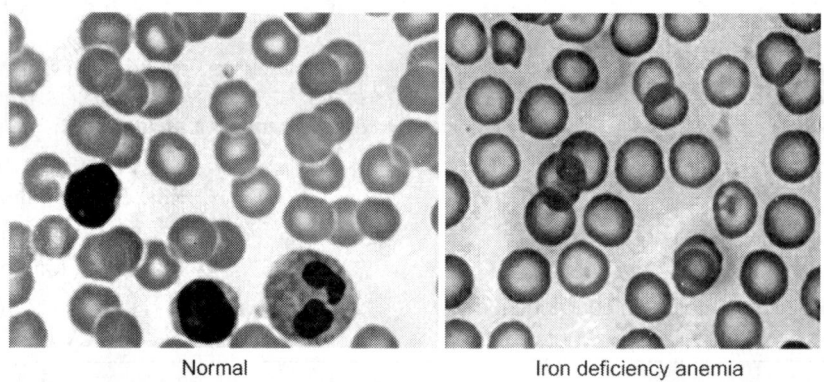

Normal   Iron deficiency anemia

Fig. 6.1: Hypochromic microcytic red blood cells. Note the enlarged central pallor in the red blood cells in iron deficiency anemia (hypochromia)

(b) Pernicious anemia

In India, pernicious anemia is not common. Pernicious anemia is caused by deficiency of vitamin B_{12} in the body. Although vitamin B_{12} content of the diet of these patients is usually normal, the vitamin is not absorbed in the gut. Normally, a glycoprotein (mol. wt. 45,000), known as **intrinsic factor**, secreted by the gastric mucosa, helps in the absorption of vitamin B_{12} in the ileum. Atrophy of gastric mucosa results in the absence of intrinsic factor, leading to malabsorption of vitamin B_{12}. Recent evidence suggests that pernicious anemia is an autoimmune disease. The auto-antibodies destroy both the parietal and chief cells of gastric mucosa (gastric atrophy). Deficiency of vitamin B_{12} produces a megaloblastic bone marrow reaction and a very severe degree of anemia. In the peripheral blood, the red cells are larger in size (macrocytes, MCV greater than 100 μ^3) but contain a normal concentration of haemoglobin (normochromic), i.e. vitamin B_{12} deficiency causes macrocytic normochromic type of anemia. Blood smear shows another two characteristic features of red cells. Firstly, the cells show a wider variation in shape, i.e. all the red cells are not circular disks, and vary in shape (poikilocytosis). Secondly, greater variation of cell size varies (4 μm to 12 μm, average 9.5 μm (anisocytosis); normal variation 6.7 to 7.7 μm, average 7.5 μm) (Fig. 6.2).

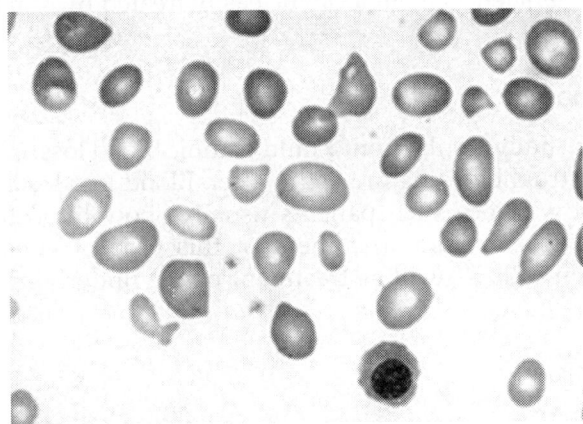

Fig. 6.2: Blood smear of a patient of pernicious anemia. Many red cells are macrocytes and there is great variation in size and shape of red cells

Neural symptoms in pernicious anemia: Vitamin B_{12} is essential for synthesis of myelin. Therefore, vitamin B_{12} deficiency results in destruction of thick myelinated fibers in central and peripheral nervous system. Therefore, besides severe anemia, deficiency of vitamin B_{12} is associated with peripheral neuropathy and degeneration of posterior and lateral white columns of spinal cord (Fig. 6.3).

Symptoms

➢ Lack of coordination
➢ Pain, numbness, and tingling in hands or feet
➢ Sensory loss
➢ Weakness of muscles

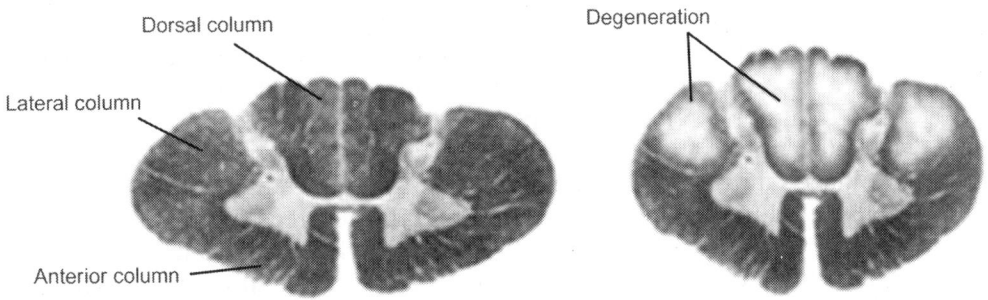

Fig. 6.3: Degeneration of white columns of spinal cord in a patient of pernicious anemia (right). Compare with normal (left)

The disorder, if not treated, is invariably fatal. Pernicious anemia can be treated by regular administration of vitamin B_{12} by intramuscular route.

(c) Folic acid deficiency anemia

It occurs in individuals who do not take enough of folic acid-rich food (green leafy vegetables, fresh fruits, meat). Folic acid deficiency is fairly common during pregnancy. It produces macrocytic normochromic type of anemia but there are no neurological problems. Folic acid deficiency anemia can be easily treated by oral administration of folic acid.

2. Hemorrhagic Anemia

This type of anemia usually results from a mild chronic blood loss, e.g. due to bleeding piles, excessive menstrual bleeding or gastric ulcer. Blood loss leads to excessive loss of iron from the body. Hence such patients usually show hypochromic microcytic (iron deficiency) type of anemia. Treatment of this type of anemia involves oral administration of iron salts as well as treatment of the underlying cause of chronic blood loss.

3. Hemolytic Anemia

The lifespan of normal red blood cells is approximately 120 days. Due to various congenital or acquired defects in the red blood cells, the life span of the red cells may be markedly reduced (as low as 30 days). The bone marrow tries to compensate for increased rate of red cell destruction by accelerated rate of erythropoiesis. When the rate of red cell regeneration cannot keep pace with the rate of red cell destruction, **anemia** develops. Moreover, increased rate of red cell destruction overloads the excretory pathways of haemoglobin degradation products (bilirubin). **Jaundice** (hemolytic type) develops when the rate of bilirubin production exceeds the bilirubin excretory capacity of the liver. Hemolytic anemia is usually normocytic normochromic type since there is no nutritional deficiency. Congenital hemolytic anemia is fairly common in India.

Causes

A. **Congenital hemolytic anemia**
  i. *Congenital (hereditary) spherocytosis:* This disorder is caused by a congenital defect in the structural proteins in cell membrane of red cells. Two important proteins, namely, spectrin and ankyrin, maintain the normal shape of red blood cells. A genetic defect in the synthesis of either of the two proteins results in reduced surface area to volume ratio of the red cells. The cells tend to attain a spherical shape. Spherical shape makes the red cells less flexible. Spherocytes cannot bend or twist during passage through narrow capillaries and hence are damaged. The spleen seems to possess a special ability to detect and trap even mildly damaged red cells. Greater red cell destruction causes enlargement of spleen. Thus, besides haemolytic anemia, splenomegaly is an important clinical feature of this disorder. The defect is inherited as an autosomal dominant trait.
  ii. *Congenital disorders of hemoglobin:* Hemolytic anemia may be due to a congenital defect in the globin chains of hemoglobin. These defects can mainly be divided into:
      (a) The hemoglobinopathies when there is an alteration in the amino acid sequences of a polypeptide chain of hemoglobin, e.g. Hb S, Hb C, Hb D.

(b) The thalassemia in which the amino acid sequence is not disturbed but synthesis of one of the two types of chains (α or β) is impaired.

In the hemoglobinopathies, the altered amino acid sequence results in an abnormality in the solubility of haemoglobin. Consequently, there is a striking abnormality in red cell morphology, which renders the red cell more prone to hemolysis, especially in the spleen.

In thalassemia, suppression of either α or β chains results in deficient haemoglobin synthesis. Moreover, absence of one type of polypeptide chain results in excessive production of the other type. This results in a disturbance in hemoglobin solubility and hence excessive hemolysis.

(a) Sickle cell anemia: This hemoglobinopathy is caused by the presence of amino acid valine instead of glutamic acid at position 6 of the β chains of haemoglobin. This variant is known as haemoglobin S (Hb S), because when deoxygenated, it polymerizes and distorts the red cell membrane into a sickle shape or a crescent shape (Fig. 6.4). Hb S is highly prevalent in the black population of Africa, but may be found in other countries also. Sickle cell anemia occurs in those individuals who are homozygous for Hb S gene. In such patients the entire haemoglobin is Hb S type. In individuals who are heterozygous for Hb S gene, the red cells contain Hb S (50%) as well as normal Hb A (50%). Such individuals are said to have sickle cell trait. They act as carriers for the abnormal gene but do not suffer from hemolytic anemia.

The sickle cells are not only abnormal in shape but also less elastic than normal biconcave red cells. The abnormal morphology makes the sickle cells more prone to haemolysis as well as gives a tendency to block the capillaries. The resultant tissue hypoxia causes further sickling of the red cells.

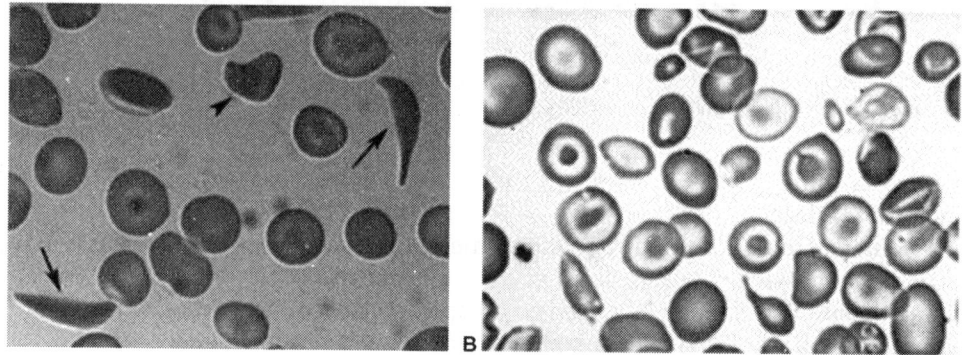

A   B

Fig. 6.4: (A) Blood smear of a patient with sickle cell anemia (sickled cells marked with arrows) (B) Blood smear of a patient with thalassemia

(b) The Thalassemia: In thalassemia, basic defect is under-production of one type of the chains of globin component of haemoglobin. Two types of thalassemia are known: Thalassemia α and thalassemia β, depending on the name of the under-produced chains. In either case, the condition may be homozygous (thalassemia major) or heterozygous (thalassemia minor). Beta-thalassemia is common in Mediterranean region, whereas α thalassemia is seen in south-east Asia including India. Anemia is mild in patients with thalassemia minor, but very severe in those with thalassemia major. In the deficiency of one type of polypeptide chain, the red cells develop the tetramers of the other type, making red cells more prone to hemolysis.

B. **Acquired haemolytic anemia:** Acquired hemolytic anemia results from development of auto-antibodies against red cells of the patient resulting in excessive destruction of the red cells. The auto-antibodies formed against red cell membrane antigens cause inappropriate destruction of red cells. Such type of anemia is not common in India.

4. Aplastic Anemia

Complete cessation of erythropoiesis is rare but very serious and often fatal type of anemia. It arises as a complication of hypersensitivity reaction to certain drugs, e.g. chloramphenicol, sulfonamides, etc. Excessive irradiation and cytotoxic drugs used in the treatment of malignant disorders also depress the bone marrow. In most of such cases, besides very severe anemia, severe leucopenia and thrombocytopenia is also present. Death may occur due to infection or severe blood loss. Bone marrow examination reveals presence of adipose tissue where red bone marrow is normally present (Fig. 6.5B) indicating cessation of hemopoiesis.

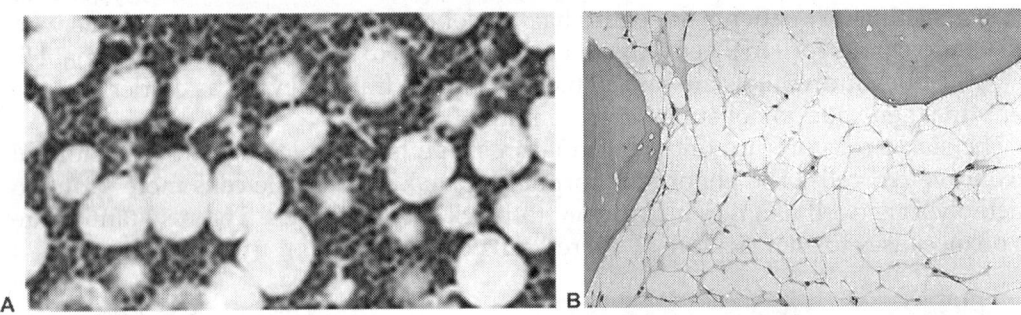

Fig. 6.5: Bone marrow (A) Normal; (B) in a patient with aplastic anemia

Complications of Anemia

Left untreated, anemia can cause many health problems, such as:
➢ **Severe fatigue:** Severe anemia can make you so tired that you cannot complete everyday tasks.
➢ **Pregnancy complications:** Pregnant women with folate deficiency anemia may be more likely to have complications, such as premature birth.
➢ **Heart problems:** Anemia can lead to a rapid or irregular heartbeat (arrhythmia). Severe anemia can lead to an enlarged heart or heart failure.
➢ **Death:** Some inherited anemias, such as sickle cell anemia, can lead to life-threatening complications.

◁ BLEEDING DISORDERS ▷

When a blood vessel is injured, hemostasis (stoppage of bleeding) occurs in two stages: Primary hemostasis results in formation of platelet plug which stops bleeding temporarily. Next step, secondary hemostasis results in clotting of blood which stops bleeding permanently (Fig. 6.6). Bleeding disorder may be due to a defect in either stage. Accordingly, bleeding disorders can be broadly classified into two categories:
   i. Purpura results from a defect in primary hemostasis.
   ii. Hemophilia results from a congenital defect in secondary hemostasis.

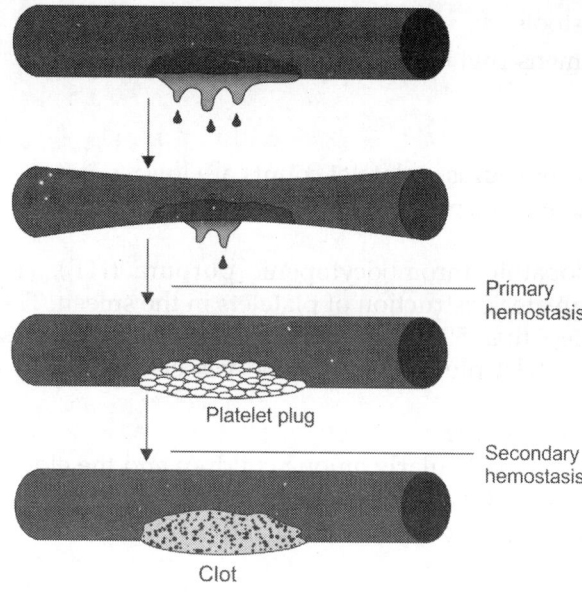

Fig. 6.6: Two-step process of hemostasis

PURPURA

Symptoms: This bleeding disorder is characterized by easy bruisability and spontaneous multiple hemorrhages under the skin and mucous membranes. At an early stage, the patient may present with numerous red spots of the size of pinhead on the skin and mucous membranes (petechial hemorrhages). In more severe form, there are larger bleeding spots (Fig. 6.7A)
➤ Easy or excessive bruising
➤ Superficial bleeding into the skin that appears as pinpoint-sized reddish-purple spots (petechiae)
➤ Bleeding from the gums or nose

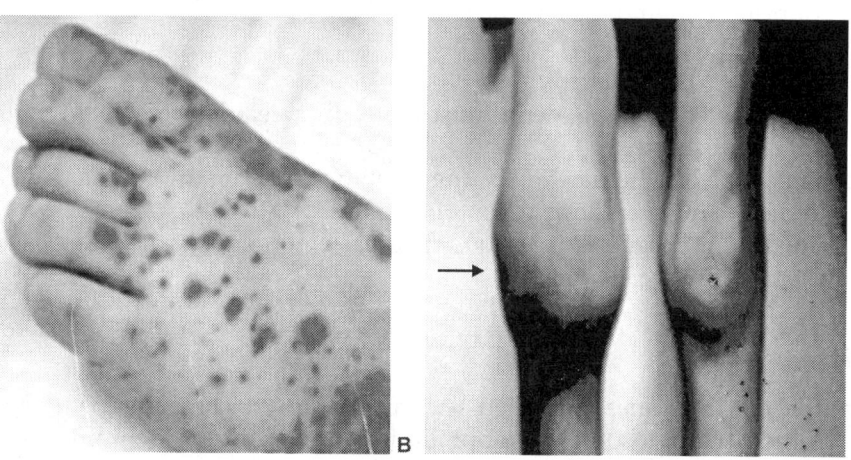

Fig. 6.7: (A) Purpura; (B) Hemarthrosis in hemophilia

➤ Blood in urine or stools
➤ Unusually heavy menstrual flow

Aetiology

➤ Thrombocytopenic purpuras—platelet counts are low.
➤ Nonthrombocytopenic purpuras—platelet levels are normal, suggesting another cause.

Pathogenesis: Idiopathic thrombocytopenic purpura (ITP), is an auto-immune disease resulting in greater destruction of platelets in the spleen. The platelet count in the blood is usually less than $50,000/\mu^3$. Decreased platelet count results in deficiency in the formation of platelet plugs. Hence blood vessels leak blood spontaneously or on mild trauma.

Risk factors for purpura include:

➤ Infectious diseases, particularly among children and the elderly
➤ Poor nutrition when it leads to a lack of vitamin C
➤ Some forms of cancer, such as leukemia and myeloma
➤ Advanced age
➤ Poor blood vessel health

HEMOPHILIA

Symptoms: In this disorder, bleeding occurs several hours after an injury. Such bleeding mostly occurs in deep tissues like muscles and joints. Characteristic clinical findings are hemarthrosis (bleeding into a joint) (Fig. 6.7B) and muscle hematomas.

Aetiology: Hemophilia is a congenital bleeding disorder. Most commonly, there is congenital deficiency of clotting factor VIII. The condition is called hemophilia-A. In a few cases, clotting factor IX is deficient (hemophilia-B). The disorder is transmitted as X-chromosome-linked recessive trait. The only effective therapy is intravenous injections of the deficient clotting factor.

Pathogenesis. Factors VIII and IX are involved in the intrinsic system of coagulation of blood. Deficiency of clotting factor VIII or IX results in formation of a weak blood clot in an injured blood vessel. Therefore, the blood vessel starts bleeding again after the effect of primary hemostasis wanes.

Complications

➤ Deep internal bleeding, e.g. deep-muscle bleeding, leading to swelling, numbness or pain of a limb.
➤ Joint damage from hemarthrosis (hemophilic arthropathy), with severe pain, disfigurement, and even destruction of the joint.
➤ Intracranial hemorrhage is a serious medical emergency which can cause brain damage and death.

Genetics

The X and Y chromosomes are called sex chromosomes. The gene for hemophilia is carried on the X chromosome. Hemophilia is inherited in an X-chromosome linked recessive manner. Females inherit two X chromosomes, one from their mother and one from their father (XX). Males inherit an X chromosome from their mother and a

Y chromosome from their father (XY). That means if a son inherits an X chromosome carrying hemophilia from his mother, he will suffer from hemophilia. It also means that fathers cannot pass hemophilia on to their sons.

But because daughters have two X chromosomes, even if they inherit the hemophilia gene from their mother, most likely they will inherit a healthy X chromosome from their father and not have hemophilia. A daughter who inherits an X chromosome that contains the gene for hemophilia is called a carrier. She can pass the gene on to her children. Hemophilia can occur in daughters, but is rare.

For a female carrier, there are four possible outcomes for each pregnancy (Fig. 6.8):
1. A girl who is not a carrier
2. A girl who is a carrier
3. A boy without hemophilia
4. A boy with hemophilia

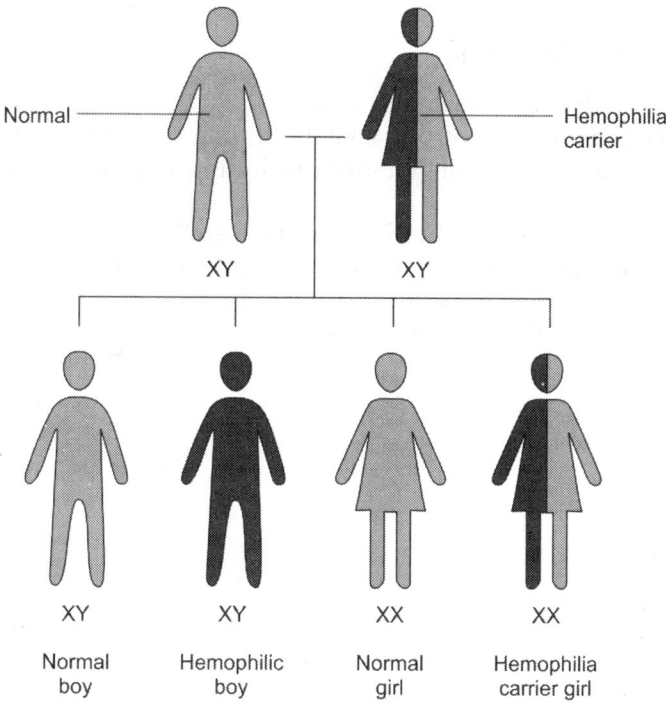

Fig. 6.8: Genetics of hemophilia

Spontaneous mutations of gene account for about 30% of all cases of hemophilia, i.e. family history may be absent.

Acquired Defects of Secondary Hemostasis

These defects are far more common than congenital disorders of secondary hemostasis. Clotting factors prothrombin (clotting factor II) and clotting factors VII, IX and X are synthesised in the liver. Their synthetic reactions requires vitamin K (Fig. 6.9). Severe liver disease or deficiency of vitamin K may cause deficiency of these clotting factors leading to severe and prolonged bleeding after a minor trauma. Intestinal bleeding is one of the serious complications of liver cirrhosis.

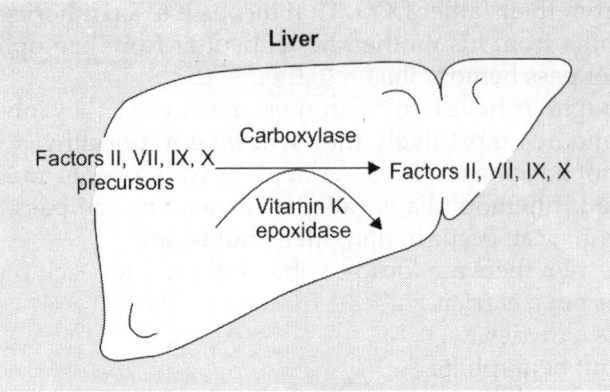

Fig. 6.9: Synthesis of clotting factors in the liver

Causes of Vitamin K Deficiency

1. Some newborn babies are vitamin K deficient.
2. Obstructive jaundice: Since bile containing bile salts does not reach the small intestine, fats and fat soluble vitamins including vitamin K are not absorbed in the gut.
3. Prolonged administration of broad-spectrum antibiotics destroys bacteria in the large intestine. These bacteria are an important source of vitamin K.
4. Overdose of oral anticoagulants (dicoumarol)
5. Dietary deficiency of vitamin K is rare.

Endocrine Disorders

<DIABETES MELLITUS>

Diabetes currently affects more than 62 million Indians, which is more than 7.2% of the adult population. Nearly 1 million Indians die due to diabetes every year. The high incidence is attributed to a combination of genetic susceptibility plus adoption of a high-calorie diet, coupled with low-activity lifestyle by India's growing middle class. Two types of diabetes mellitus (DM) are recognised:

TYPE I DM

Type I or insulin-dependent diabetes mellitus (IDDM) is juvenile-onset diabetes. In type I diabetes, there is an absolute deficiency of insulin. It is believed to be an autoimmune disease, which manifests in childhood. The patients are usually lean. Ketosis and acidosis are common complications of this type of diabetes. Plasma insulin levels are very low or undetectable.

TYPE II DM

Type II diabetes manifests after the age of 40 years. Most of the patients with this type of diabetes are obese. Plasma insulin levels are often normal or even elevated. But, there seems to be a deficiency of insulin receptors in the tissues so that at tissue level, circulating insulin is ineffective. Ketotic-acidosis is not very common in type II diabetes.

Symptoms and Signs of DM
➢ Polyuria
➢ Polydipsia
➢ Weight loss despite polyphagia
➢ Hyperglycemia
➢ Glycosuria
➢ Muscle weakness
➢ Frequent infections

➤ Ketosis
➤ Acidosis and
➤ Coma

▌PATHOGENESIS

At metabolic level, fundamental defects in DM are:
➤ Decreased glucose utilization
➤ Increased glucose production
➤ Increased lipolysis
➤ Increased protein catabolism

Diabetes mellitus starts without any symptoms. Gradually, the condition worsens and when blood sugar level is above 180 mg%, sugar appears in the urine. Only then the patient may become aware of the problem. In many cases, diabetic patients come to know about their disease only when they visit a physician for some other ailment and blood glucose level is tested.

1. Hyperglycemia and its Consequences

Hyperglycemia is one of the cardinal features of diabetes mellitus. It is due to (i) decreased peripheral utilization of glucose and (ii) increased hepatic production of glucose (gluconeogenesis). Mild transient hyperglycemia is harmless and occurs after every meal. But when the blood glucose level is chronically elevated, numerous complications arise. When the blood glucose level exceeds the renal threshold, glucose appears in the urine (**glycosuria**) (Fig. 7.1).

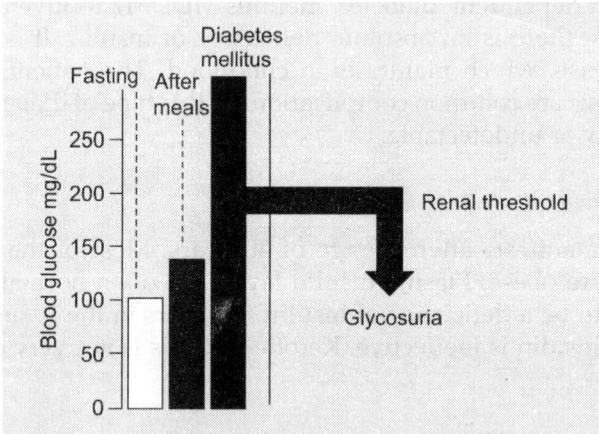

Fig. 7.1: Glycosuria occurs only when the blood sugar level exceeds the renal threshold for glucose

Renal excretion of osmotically active glucose molecules leads to the loss of large amount of water in the urine (osmotic diuresis). The resultant dehydration activates the thirst mechanism leading to large amount of water intake (**polydipsia**). The loss of glucose in the urine means loss of energy (calories) from the body. Appreciable amount of Na^+ and K^+ are lost in the urine as side effects of osmotic diuresis. Deficient utilization of glucose in the hypothalamic ventromedial nuclei (satiety center) causes **hyperphagia**. In spite of excessive food intake, there is a **loss of the body weight** because of loss of calories in the urine and mobilization of fats and proteins for energy production.

Hyperglycemia impairs all aspects of leucocyte phagocytic function: Adherence, diapedesis, phagocytosis and intracellular killing. Therefore diabetic patients are more liable to infections.

Chronically elevated blood glucose level results in attachment of glucose (glycosylation) of hemoglobin and tissue proteins. Tissue protein damage is responsible for long-term complication such as neuropathy, retinopathy, cataract, and nephropathy (kidney damage) and hypertension (Fig. 7.2).

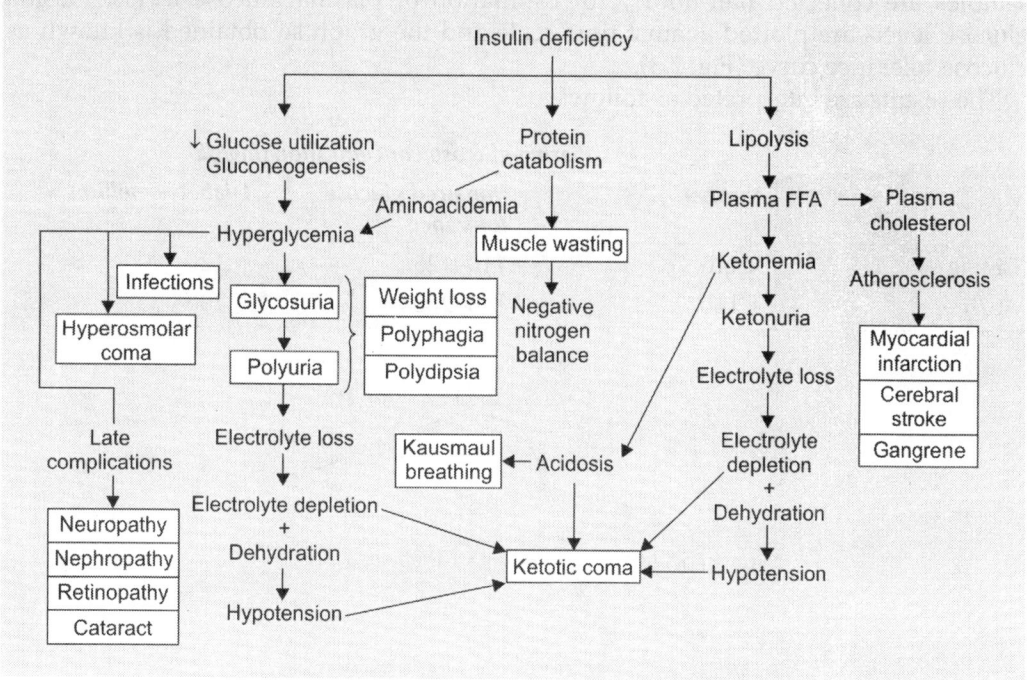

Fig. 7.2: Pathophysiology of diabetes mellitus

2. Ketosis and its Consequences (Fig. 7.2)

Deficiency of insulin causes great reduction in lipogenesis and accelerates the process of lipolysis. As a result, plasma level of FFA is more than doubled.

Free fatty acids provide energy to the glucose-starved insulin-sensitive tissues, like skeletal muscle. However, FFA mobilization also causes formation of ketone bodies. The ketone bodies formation exceeds the rate of their utilization leading to ketosis and acidosis. Acidosis results in rapid, deep respiration (dyspnoea). Patient's breathe smells of acetone. The urine becomes highly acidic. When the capacity of kidney to replace plasma cations accompanying the organic anions with H^+ and NH_4 is exceeded, Na^+ and K^+ are lost in the urine. The electrolyte and water loss leads to dehydration, hypovolaemia and hypotension. Finally acidosis and dehydration may depress the consciousness to the level of coma and death.

Chronic hyperlipidaemia leads to atherosclerosis which causes coronary artery disease and cerebral stroke and gangrene in lower limbs.

3. Protein Catabolism (Fig. 7.2)

In diabetes, protein anabolism is suppressed and catabolism is increased. Large amount of amino acids are used for energy production. Amino acids also act as substrate for enhanced gluconeogenesis promoted by insulin deficiency. Consequently, the patient suffers from loss of weight, protein depletion, wasting and negative nitrogen balance.

Glucose Tolerance Test (GTT)

This is a test for the diagnosis of diabetes mellitus. After an overnight fast, a venous blood sample is taken. Then, the patient is given 75 g of glucose orally and four blood samples are collected half-hourly for estimation of plasma glucose levels. Plasma glucose levels are plotted against time scale and the graph so obtained is known as glucose tolerance curve (Fig. 7.3).

The results are interpreted as follows:

	Plasma glucose concentration (mg/dL)		
	Normal	*Impaired glucose tolerance*	*Diabetes mellitus*
Fasting	<110	110–125	>126
At 2h	<140	140–200	>200

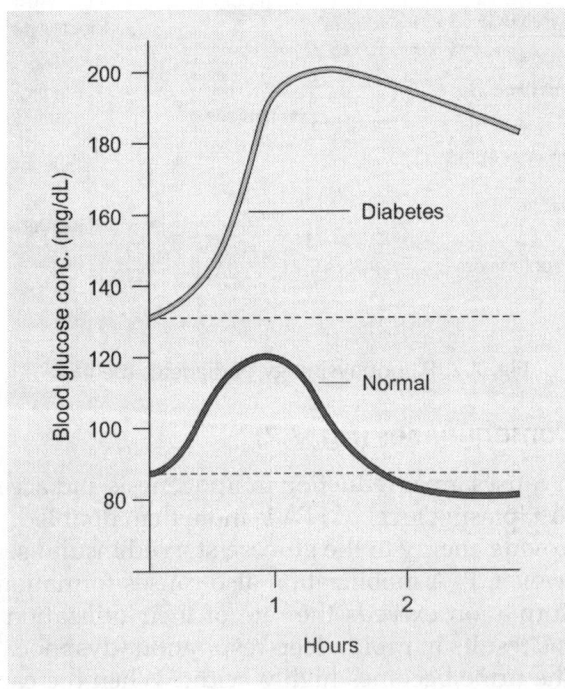

Fig. 7.3: Normal and diabetic glucose tolerance curve

Important Role of Estimation of Glycosylated Hemoglobin

In a normal subject, glucose molecules get *non-enzymic* attachment to a small proportion (<7%) of hemoglobin-A to form glycosylated hemoglobin (Fig. 7.4). In case of sustained hyperglycaemia, such as in diabetes mellitus, greater proportion (10–20%) of haemoglobin is glycosylated. The concentration of glycosylated hemoglobin has been found to reflect average blood glucose level during the previous 6–8 weeks. Therefore, its measurement has become an important tool for proper regulation of antidiabetic therapy, that is, to find out whether the given dose of the medication has been able to maintain blood glucose level within the physiological range during the previous 6–8 weeks. (Glucose tolerance test reflects the glucose level on the day of the test only.)

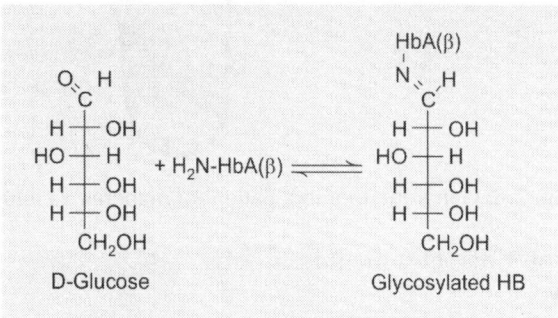

Fig. 7.4: Glycosylated hemoglobin

Long-term Complications of DM

➢ Neuropathy, leading to numbness and muscle weakness
➢ Retinopathy, leading to blindness (Fig. 7.5)
➢ Cataract
➢ Nephropathy, leading to chronic renal failure
➢ Hypertension
➢ Coronary artery disease, and
➢ Strokes.
➢ Gangrene in lower limbs (Fig. 7.6)

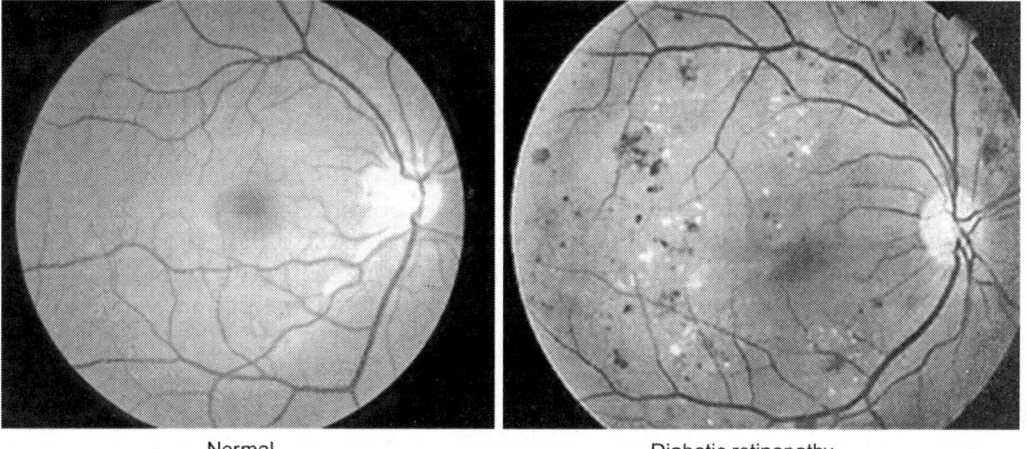

Normal   Diabetic retinopathy

Fig. 7.5: Retina, normal and in diabetic retinopathy

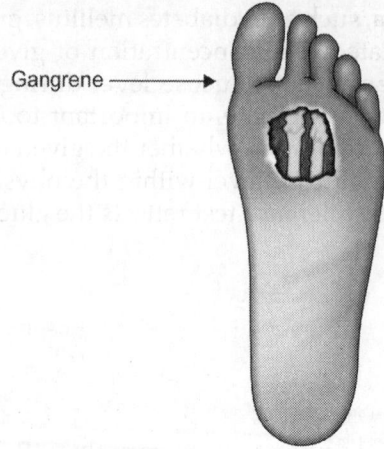

Gangrene

Fig. 7.6: Gangrene foot in a patient of diabetes mellitus

Risk factors for type 1 diabetes include:
➢ **Family history**
➢ **Genetics.** The presence of certain genes indicates an increased risk of developing type 1 diabetes.
➢ **Geography.** The incidence of type 1 diabetes tends to increase as you travel away from the equator.

Risk factors for type 2 diabetes include:
➢ **Overweight**
➢ **Inactivity**
➢ **Family history**
➢ **Age.** The risk of type 2 diabetes increases as you get older, especially after age 45.
➢ **Prediabetes.** Prediabetes is a condition in which one's blood sugar level is higher than normal, but not high enough to be classified as diabetes. Left untreated, prediabetes often progresses to type 2 diabetes.
➢ **Gestational diabetes.** If one develops gestational diabetes, she has greater risk of type 2 diabetes.

DISORDERS OF THYROID GLAND

Diseases of the thyroid gland are among the most abundant endocrine disorders worldwide second only to diabetes; India is no exception. Recent report shows that 300 million people in the world are suffering from thyroid disorders and among them about 42 million people reside in India. Hypothyroidism is the most common thyroid disorder. Hyperthyroidism is less common. Thyroid disorders are more common in women than in men.

1. HYPERTHYROIDISM

Hyperthyroidism results from excessive secretion of thyroid hormones. It is known as Graves' disease or exophthalmic goitre. Less commonly, excessive thyroxine secretion is due to a thyroid adenoma (toxic thyroid adenoma).

Aetiology

Graves' disease is an autoimmune disorder characterized by development of thyroid-stimulating immunoglobulin (TSI). TSI acts on thyroid stimulating hormone receptors (TSH-receptors) on the thyroid follicular cells to activate thyroid hormone synthesis and release as well as causes hypertrophy and increased vascularity of thyroid gland. This results in the characteristic picture of Graves' thyrotoxicosis, with a diffusely enlarged thyroid and excessive plasma thyroxine levels.

Pathology

There is a diffuse thyroid enlargement of thyroid gland (goitre). Microscopically, thyroid follicles are hypercellular and lined by tall columnar cells. In the follicles, colloid is scanty and shows semi-lunar erosions near the follicular cells. Stroma shows lymphocytic infiltration. (Fig. 7.7)

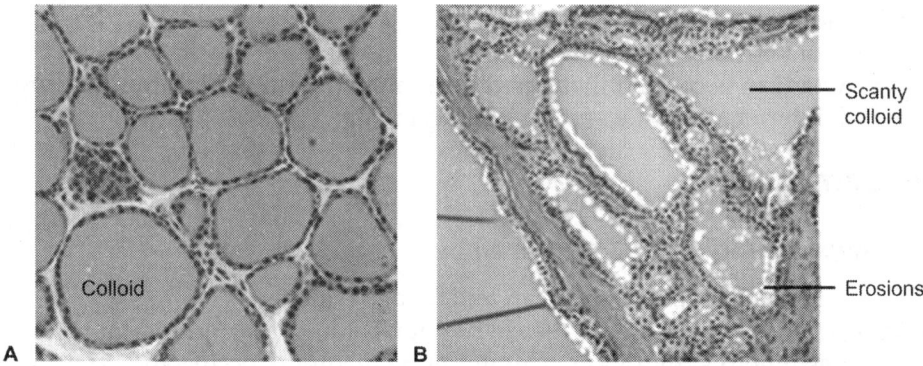

Fig. 7.7: Microscopic appearance of thyroid gland. (A) Normal; (B) hyperthyroidism

Symptoms and signs: *All the symptoms and signs reflect the effects of increased plasma thyroxine levels on various organs and tissues of the body:*
➢ Palpitation
➢ Tachycardia
➢ Nervousness
➢ Loss of weight
➢ Easy fatigability
➢ Restlessness
➢ Fine tremor
➢ Excessive appetite
➢ Diarrhea
➢ Excessive sweating
➢ Heat intolerance
➢ Muscle weakness
➢ Increased basal metabolic rate (BMR)
  Some patients develop protrusion of eyeballs due to oedematous swelling of retro-bulbar tissue (exophthalmos) (Fig. 7.8).

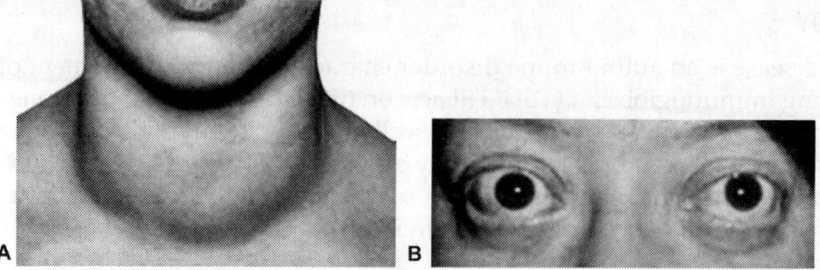

Fig. 7.8: A patient of Graves' disease. (A) Diffuse goitre; (B) exophthalmos

Complications

➢ Tachycardia
➢ Atrial fibrillation
➢ Congestive heart failure
➢ Osteoporosis
➢ Ophthalmopathy
➢ Hyperthyroid crisis

Hyperthyroidism is commonly treated by administration of anti-thyroid drugs, i.e. drugs which interfere with the synthesis of thyroxine.

2. HYPOTHYROIDISM

a. Adult Hypothyroidism (Myxoedema)

This is a common disorder especially in middle age females.

Aetiology. The most common cause of hypothyroidism is an autoimmune disorder known as Hashimoto's thyroiditis. Autoimmune disorders occur when our immune system produces antibodies that attack our own tissues.

Pathology: Microscopically, thyroid shows atrophic follicles, fibrosis and diffuse lymphocytic infiltration (Fig. 7.9).

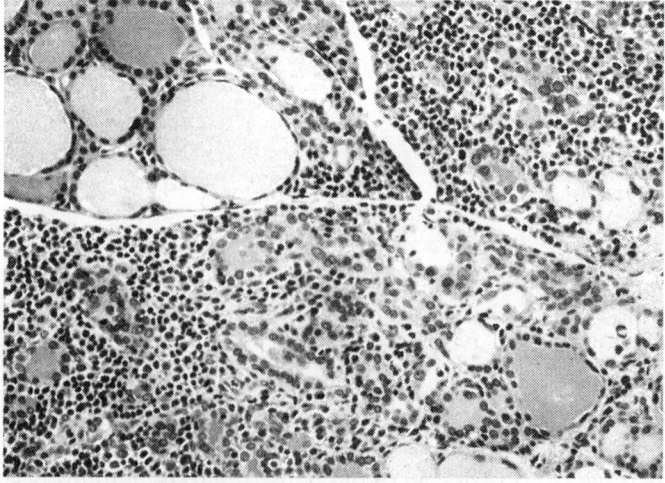

Fig. 7.9: Microscopic appearance of Hashimoto's thyroiditis

Symptoms and signs. *All the symptoms signs are the result of decreased plasma thyroxine levels on various tissues of the body.*

➢ Puffy face (Fig. 7.10) is a characteristic finding. It is due to accumulation of myxomatous gel in the subcutaneous tissue in the face.

➢ Slow heart rate
➢ Increased body weight
➢ Constipation
➢ Decreased appetite
➢ Somnolence
➢ Mental sluggishness

➢ Cold intolerance
➢ Muscle weakness
➢ Dry skin (lack of sweating)
➢ Low BMR
➢ High blood cholesterol

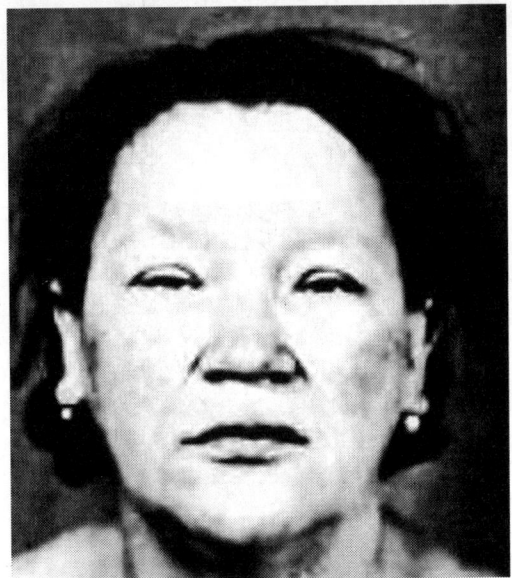

Fig. 7.10: Myxoedema

Complications

➢ Atherosclerosis
➢ Coronary artery disease
➢ Congestive heart failure
➢ Stroke
➢ Infertility
➢ Hypothermia
➢ Mental depression
➢ Myxoedema coma

Hypothyroidism is easily treated by oral administration of thyroxine.

b. Cretinism

This disorder results from congenital deficiency of thyroxine. The child's physical and mental growth is retarded leading to permanent mental deficit. The most common cause of cretinism is maternal iodine deficiency during pregnancy. By the time the typical clinical picture develops in the infant, it is usually too late to reverse the mental retardation. Realization of this fact has led to widespread use of iodised salt in India and many other countries.

c. Iodine-deficiency Goitre

Dietary intake of at least 100–150 µg of iodide per day is required for normal thyroid function. Inadequate thyroid secretion occurs when iodide intake falls below 10 µg/day. Due to negative feedback mechanism, the secretion of TSH from the anterior pituitary is increased leading to hypertrophy of the thyroid gland. The enlarged hypertrophied thyroid gland so produced is known as iodine-deficiency goitre (Fig. 7.11). Use of iodised salt can prevent the disorder.

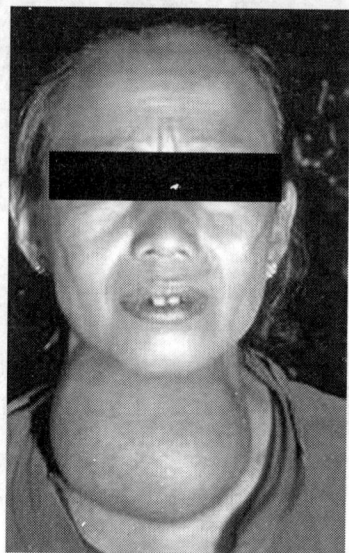

Fig. 7.11: Iodine deficiency goitre

DISORDERS OF SEX HORMONES

TESTOSTERONE DEFICIENCY

It is hard to know how many men among us have testosterone deficiency (TD), although data suggest that overall about 2.1% may have TD. As few as 1% of younger men may have TD, while as many as 50% of men over 80 years old may have TD.

Symptoms

➢ Reduced sex drive
➢ Reduced erectile function
➢ Loss of body hair
➢ Less beard growth
➢ Loss of lean muscle mass
➢ Feeling very tired all the time (fatigue)
➢ Symptoms of depression

Causes

➢ Klinefelter syndrome (rare congenital defect)
➢ Damage to testicles by accident
➢ Removal of testicles because of cancer
➢ Aging
➢ Obesity
➢ Metabolic syndrome (high blood pressure, high blood sugar, unhealthy cholesterol levels, and belly fat)
➢ Use of medications such as antidepressants and narcotic pain medications

ERECTILE DYSFUNCTION (IMPOTENCE)

Erectile dysfunction is defined as the inability to attain a penile erection of sufficient rigidity for vaginal penetration. The prevalence of impotence increases rapidly after the age of 50 years, especially in those with diabetes mellitus or atherosclerosis.

Impotence may be due to severe hypogonadism which causes erectile failure as well as loss of libido (sexual interest and initiative). However, in most of the cases, the erectile dysfunction can be attributed to atherosclerosis of the penile blood vessels or autonomic neuropathy involving nervi erigentes. In some cases, impotence may be psychological.

Infertility

The failure to conceive after one year of unprotected intercourse is called infertility. It affects about 10% of married couples. The problem may be in the husband or the wife or both. The congenital causes of male infertility are not common. More common causes of male infertility are acquired defects of the testes which include viral orchitis (mumps virus) and testicular trauma. The patient's semen usually shows low sperm count and/or decrease sperm motility.

LOW OESTROGEN LEVELS

Causes

➢ Turner syndrome
(a rare congenital defect)
➢ Premature ovarian failure
➢ Thyroid disorders
➢ Excessive exercise
➢ Being severely underweight
➢ Low-functioning pituitary gland

Symptoms

➢ Irregular periods.
➢ Infertility: Low estrogen levels can prevent ovulation and make getting pregnant difficult, leading to infertility.

Female Infertility

Absence of ovulation during the reproductive age of the female may result from isolated gonadotropin deficiency or primary ovarian failure. Blockade of fallopian tubes by pelvic inflammation is a fairly common cause of female infertility in spite of normal ovulatory ovarian cycles.

Disorders of
Nervous System

STROKE

Stroke is one of the most devastating consequence of two common diseases, atherosclerosis and hypertension. It represents the second leading cause of death (after coronary artery disease) and a major cause of disability worldwide. Besides age, hypertension is the most important cardiovascular risk factor for developing both ischemic and hemorrhagic stroke.

Definition

The sudden death of some brain cells due to lack of oxygen when the blood flow to the brain is impaired by blockage or rupture of an artery to the brain is known as stroke.

Causes

There are two types of stroke.

➢ **Ischemic stroke** In a patient with atherosclerosis, a thrombus formation in one of the blood vessels supplying the brain blocks the blood flow to a part of the brain (Fig. 8.1A). That area undergoes ischemic necrosis and loss of function. In some patients, a blood clot in the heart or a blood vessel becomes loose (called embolus), travels in the arterial system and blocks a blood vessel in the brain, resulting in ischaemia and necrosis. Ischemic stroke can also occur when a large atherosclerotic plaque clogs the brain's blood vessels. About 80% of all strokes are ischaemic.

➢ **Hemorrhagic strokes** occur when a blood vessel in the brain ruptures (Fig. 8.1B). The result is blood seeping into the brain tissue, causing damage to brain cells. The most common causes of hemorrhagic stroke are high blood pressure and cerebral artery aneurysms. An aneurysm is an abnormal focal dilation of an artery in the brain that results from a weakening of the muscular layer.

Symptoms

The most common symptoms of a stroke are:
➢ Weakness or numbness of the face, arm, or leg on one side of the body
➢ Loss of vision in one or both eyes

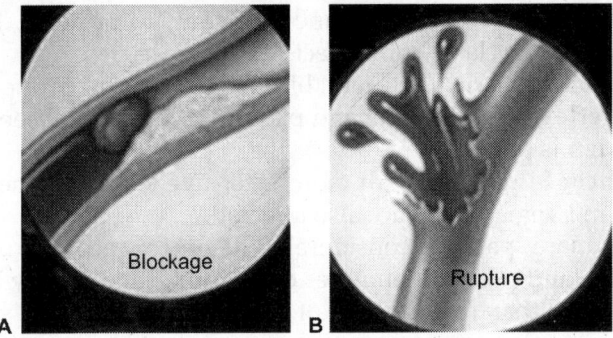

Fig. 8.1: Types of stroke. (A) Ischemic and (B) hemorrhagic

➤ Loss of speech, difficulty talking, or understanding what others are saying
➤ Sudden, severe headache
➤ Loss of balance or unstable walking

Signs

1. **Paralysis:** The paralysis affects movements of the face, arm and leg (Fig. 8.2)

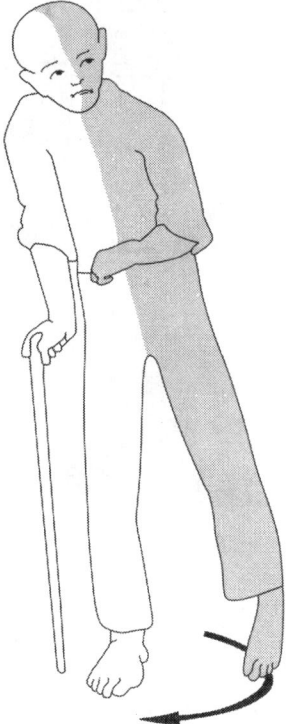

Fig. 8.2: A patient with left-sided hemiplegia

2. **Muscle tone:** Hypertonia (spasticity) is most prominent in the antigravity muscles (flexors of the upper limb and extensors of the lower limb). When a passive flexion of a limb is attempted, initially the examiner feels lot of resistance. But if

the attempt is continued, the resistance suddenly disappears. This phenomenon is called spasticity or clasp-knife effect.

3. **Deep reflexes:** Knee jerk, ankle jerk, biceps jerk are exaggerated.
4. **Superficial reflexes:** Abdominal and plantar reflexes are absent.
5. **Babinski's sign** is present.
6. **Sensory deficit:** In patients with more extensive lesions of the internal capsule, the sensory and visual fibers are also affected.
7. **Recovery:** In many patients considerable degree of recovery occurs. Muscles of the lower limb and proximal muscles of the upper limb show better recovery of voluntary control than fine muscles of the hands and fingers.

Pathogenesis

a. Ischemic Stroke

Ischemic stroke occurs because of a loss of blood supply to part of the brain. Cerebral ischemia initiates a series of changes called the ischemic cascade. Brain tissue ceases to function if deprived of oxygen for more than 60 to 90 seconds, and after approximately three hours will suffer irreversible injury leading to the death of the tissue, i.e. cerebral infarction (Fig. 8.3).

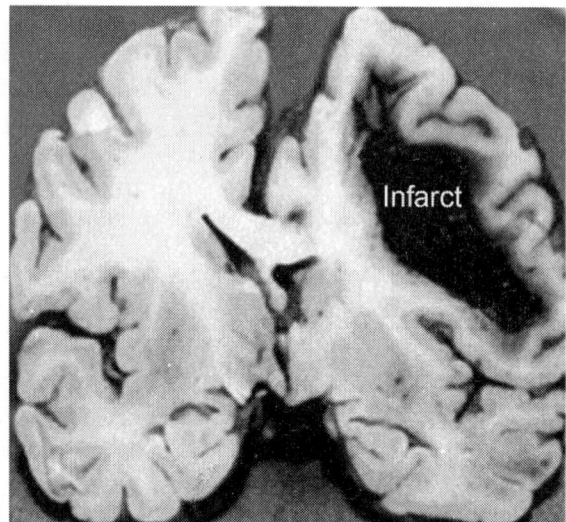

Fig. 8.3: Cerebral infarct

Atherosclerosis may disrupt the blood supply by (i) narrowing the lumen of blood vessels leading to a reduction of blood flow, or (ii) by causing the formation of blood clots within the vessel. (iii) Embolic infarction occurs when emboli formed elsewhere in the circulatory system, typically in the heart as a consequence of atrial fibrillation, or in the carotid arteries, break off, enter the cerebral circulation, then lodge in and block brain blood vessels. Brain tissue is especially vulnerable to ischaemia since it has little respiratory reserve and is completely dependent on aerobic metabolism, unlike most other organs.

Since blood vessels in the brain are now blocked, the brain becomes low in energy, and thus it resorts to using anaerobic metabolism within the region of brain tissue affected by ischemia. Anaerobic metabolism of glucose can produce adenosine triphosphate (ATP) but releases a by-product called lactic acid. Lactic acid is an irritant which could potentially destroy cells since it is an acid and disrupts the normal acid–base balance in the brain.

As oxygen or glucose becomes depleted in ischemic brain tissue, the production of ATP fails, leading to failure of energy-dependent sodium-potassium pump necessary for tissue cell survival. This sets off a series of interrelated events that result in cellular injury and death.

Besides failure of sodium–potassium pump, another major cause of neuronal injury is the release of the excitatory neurotransmitter glutamate. Glutamate is normally stored within the neurons. During neuronal activity, glutamate is released into the cerebral extracellular fluid (ECF), but its extracellular concentration is immediately decreased by its re-uptake into the neurons. The re-uptake process is also dependent on ATP-dependent sodium–potassium pump. In the deficiency of ATP, glutamate concentration in the cerebral ECF increases. Glutamate producing an influx of calcium into the neurons which activates enzymes that digest the cells' proteins, lipids, and nuclear material. Calcium influx can also lead to the failure of mitochondria, which can lead further toward energy depletion and triggers cell death. Ischemia also induces production of oxygen free radicals and other reactive oxygen species which are lethal to the neurons.

b. Hemorrhagic Strokes

Hemorrhagic stroke constitutes about 10% of total strokes. Hypertension is the major cause of rupture of a cerebral blood vessel. Rupture of an aneurysm in the cerebral artery is another cause. Hemorrhagic strokes result in mechanical tissue injury by causing compression of tissue from an expanding hematoma. In addition, the pressure may lead to a loss of blood supply to affected tissue with resulting infarction. The third pathogenic mechanism is direct toxic effect of blood in the cerebral ECF. Inflammation contributes to the secondary brain injury after hemorrhage.

Pathophysiology

The changes in the brain described above occur most often in the middle cerebral artery, which supplies the region called internal capsule. All the descending motor fibres of corticospinal tract as well as the sensory fibers ascending to sensory cortex pass through the internal capsule. Depending on the extent of lesion in the internal capsule, stroke may result in only motor deficit or motor as well as sensory deficit. Moreover, because of decussation of corticospinal tract and sensory tract in the medulla, internal capsule lesion produces motor and sensory effects on the contralateral side (Fig. 8.4). It means, if the lesion is in left internal capsule, motor and sensory deficit would occur on the right side of the body.

Risk factors

➤ High blood pressure
➤ Cigarette smoking
➤ High cholesterol
➤ Diabetes
➤ **Age**: People age 55 or older have a higher risk of stroke than do younger people
➤ **Sex**: Men have a higher risk of stroke than women.

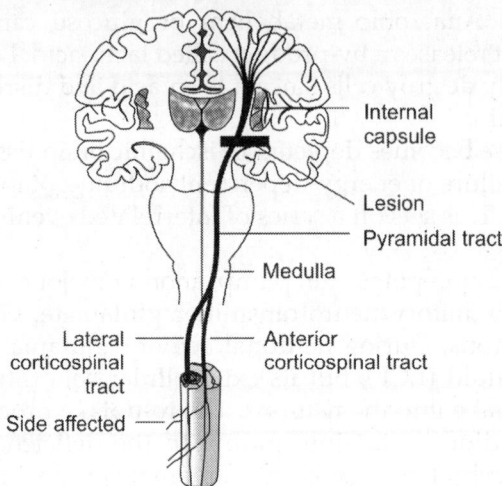

Fig. 8.4: A lesion in the internal capsule on the left side results in motor deficit on the right side of the body.

Complications

➢ Paralysis or loss of muscle movement may persist permanently
➢ Difficulty talking or swallowing may persist
➢ Memory loss or thinking difficulties.
➢ Emotional problems. Patient may develop depression.
➢ Pain.
➢ Bedsores

PARKINSON'S DISEASE

Parkinson's disease (PD) affects 1% of the population above 60 years age. It is a long-term degenerative disorder of the central nervous system that mainly affects the motor system. PD usually begins around age 60, but it can start earlier. It is more common in men than in women.

Aetiology

PD is caused by degeneration of dopaminergic neurons in the substantia nigra, one of the basal ganglia (Fig. 8.5). The cause of degeneration is not known.

Symptoms and Signs

1. **Bradykinesia:** This term is used to describe the inability to initiate movements. Poverty of movement is the most characteristic feature of Parkinson disease. The patient has *mask-like facial expression* and an *unblinking reptilian stare*. There is *absence* of normal associated movements, e.g. *swinging of the arms* during walking or change of *facial expression* related to the emotional content of the speech. Even ordinary motor tasks are performed very slowly, taking much longer time than average normal. Bradykinesia/akinesia are not due to any paralysis. Sensory system is also normal. Still there is great difficulty in initiating voluntary movements. Muscle power is not affected.

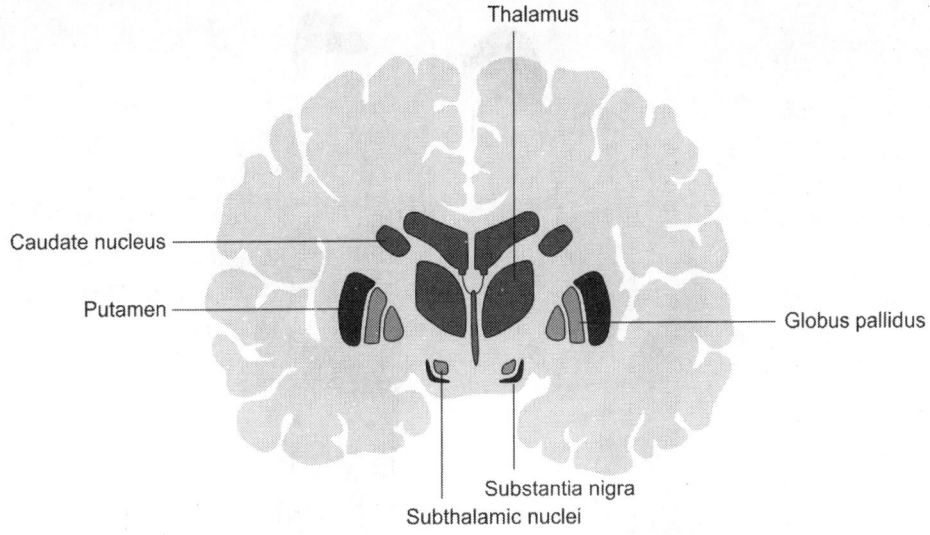

Fig. 8.5: The thalamus and basal ganglia

2. **Lead pipe rigidity:** Rigidity mostly involves the proximal muscles of the limbs. It affects both the protagonists and antagonists. During passive movement of a limb, the resistance is observed throughout the effort as if a lead pipe is being bent (i.e. there is no clasp-knife effect that is seen in patients of hemiplegia) (Fig. 8.6). When limbs of the person with PD are passively moved by the examiner, a "cogwheel rigidity" may be seen. Cogwheel-like rigidity is said to exist when a muscle is passive moved, it resists at first, but with enough force, it is partially moved until it resists again, and only with further force, will it be moved (Fig. 8.6). In advanced cases, the rigidity may increase to such an extent that the patient with arms adducted and flexed, knees flexed and the back bent has a *statue-like appearance* (Fig. 8.7).

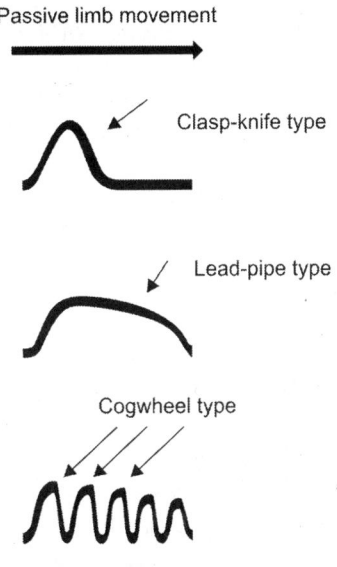

Fig. 8.6: Types of rigidity

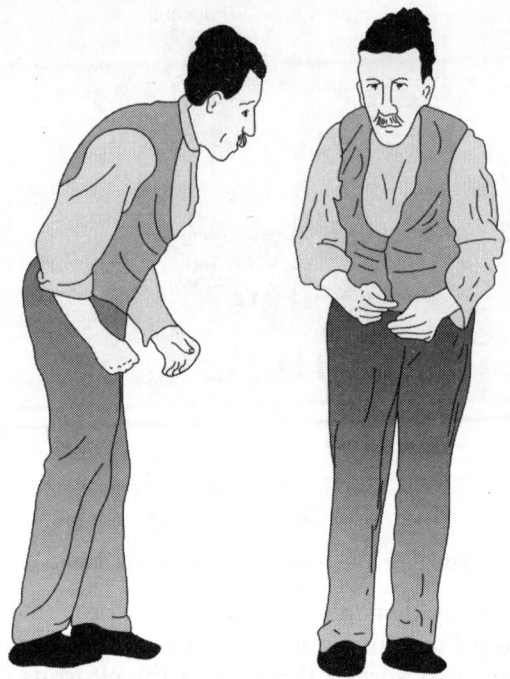

Fig. 8.7: Statue-like appearance in Parkinsonism

3. **Tremor:** Involuntary rhythmic oscillatory movements of the distal parts of the limb or the head are called tremor. Tremor are produced by alternating contraction of the protagonist and antagonist muscles. It is a pronation-supination tremor that is described as 'pill-rolling', that is the index finger of the hand tends to get into contact with the thumb, and they perform a circular movement together (Fig. 8.8). Such term was given due to the similarity of the movement in PD patients with the former pharmaceutical technique of manually making pills. Parkinsonian tremor occurs at a frequency of 4–6/s. Parkinsonian tremors are *present at rest* but disappear during sleep or voluntary activity, hence often called *resting tremor*. A patient showing severe tremor of the hand would hold a cup of tea and drink without difficulty. Parkinsonian tremor also disappear during sleep.

As mentioned above, Parkinson disease is due to degeneration of dopamine producing neurons of the substantia nigra. As a result, there is a disturbance of

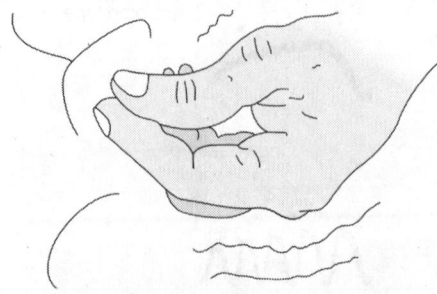

Fig. 8.8: Pill-rolling tremor

neural balance between the excitatory cholinergic and inhibitory dopaminergic activity of the neostriatum.

4. **Postural disturbance:** A forward-flexed posture (Fig. 8.7).
5. **Postural instability:** In the late stages, postural instability is typical, which leads to impaired balance and frequent falls, that may lead to bone fractures.
6. **Gait:** Shuffling gait is characterized by short steps, with feet barely leaving the ground. Small obstacles tend to cause the patient to trip.

Risk Factors

Risk factors for Parkinson's disease include:
➢ **Age:** Young adults rarely experience Parkinson's disease. It ordinarily begins in middle or late life, and the risk increases with age. People usually develop the disease around age 60 or older.
➢ **Heredity:** Having a close relative with Parkinson's disease increases the chances that you will develop the disease.
➢ **Sex:** Men are more likely to develop Parkinson's disease than are women.

Complications

Parkinson's disease is often accompanied by these additional problems:
➢ Dementia.
➢ Depression.
➢ Swallowing problems.
➢ Chewing and eating problems. Late-stage Parkinson's disease affects the muscles in the mouth, making chewing difficult.
➢ Sleep disorders.
➢ Bladder problems. Parkinson's disease may cause bladder problems, including being unable to control urine or having difficulty urinating.
➢ Constipation. Many people with Parkinson's disease develop constipation.

EPILEPSY

Epilepsy is a disorder of the brain characterized by **repeated seizures**. A seizure is defined as a sudden alteration of behavior due to a temporary change in the electrical functioning of the brain. Around 50 million people worldwide have epilepsy making it one of the most common neurological diseases globally. Nearly 80% of people with epilepsy live in low- and middle-income countries. The prevalence in India is about 1% of the population.

Symptoms and signs

Because epilepsy is caused by abnormal activity in the brain, seizures can affect any process your brain coordinates. Seizure signs and symptoms may include:
➢ Temporary confusion
➢ A staring spell
➢ Uncontrollable jerking movements of the arms and legs
➢ Loss of consciousness or awareness
➢ Psychic symptoms such as fear, anxiety

Pathogenesis

In epileptic seizures a group of neurons begin firing in an abnormal, excessive, and synchronized manner, which can be detected by electroencephalography (Fig. 8.7).

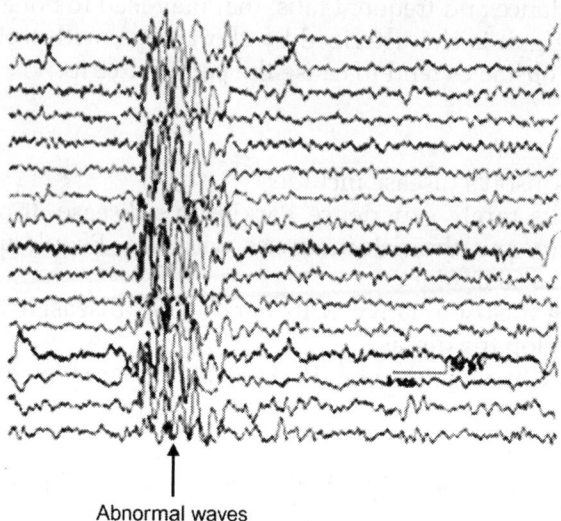

Abnormal waves

Fig. 8.9: Electroencephalogram (EEG) in epilepsy.

Causes

Epilepsy has no identifiable cause in about half the people with the condition. In the other half, the condition may be traced to various factors, including:
➤ **Genetic influence.** Some types of epilepsy run in families. In these cases, it is likely that there is a genetic influence.
➤ Brain damage from prenatal or perinatal causes (e.g. a loss of oxygen or trauma during birth, low birth weight);
➤ Congenital abnormalities or genetic conditions with associated brain malformations;
➤ A severe head injury;
➤ Stroke
➤ An infection of the brain such as meningitis, encephalitis
➤ A brain tumor.

Complications

Having a seizure at certain times can lead to circumstances that are dangerous to self or others.
➤ Falling leading to bone fractures
➤ Drowning while swimming
➤ Car accidents while driving

PSYCHIATRIC DISORDERS

Mental illness, also called mental health disorders, refers to a wide range of mental health conditions—disorders that affect your mood, thinking and behavior. Examples of mental illness include depression, anxiety disorders, schizophrenia, dementia, etc. According to WHO, globally about 25% of population suffers from some psychiatric disorder in their lifetime.

DEPRESSION

Depression is a common mental disorder and one of the main causes of disability worldwide. Globally, an estimated 264 million people are affected by depression. More women are affected than men.

Depression is characterized by sadness, loss of interest or pleasure, feelings of guilt or low self-worth, disturbed sleep or appetite, tiredness, and poor concentration. People with depression may also have multiple physical complaints with no apparent physical cause. Depression can be long-lasting or recurrent, substantially impairing people's ability to function at work or school and to cope with daily life. At its most severe, depression can lead to suicide.

Symptoms

➤ Feelings of sadness, tearfulness, emptiness or hopelessness.
➤ Angry outbursts, irritability or frustration.
➤ Loss of interest or pleasure in most or all normal activities, such as sex, hobbies or sports.
➤ Sleep disturbances, including insomnia or sleeping too much.
➤ Tiredness and lack of energy, so even small tasks take extra effort.
➤ Reduced appetite and weight loss or increased cravings for food and weight gain.
➤ Anxiety, agitation or restlessness.
➤ Slowed thinking, speaking or body movements.
➤ Feelings of worthlessness or guilt, fixating on past failures or self-blame.
➤ Trouble thinking, concentrating, making decisions and remembering things.
➤ Frequent or recurrent thoughts of death, suicidal thoughts, suicide attempts or suicide.
➤ Unexplained physical problems, such as back pain or headaches.

Causes

It is not known exactly what causes depression. As with many mental disorders, a variety of factors may be involved, such as:
➤ **Biological differences:** People with depression appear to have physical changes in their brains.
➤ **Brain chemistry:** Neurotransmitters are naturally occurring brain chemicals that likely play a role in depression. A deficiency of a neurotransmitter may lead to depression. Treatment consists of increasing concentrations of certain neurotransmitters in the brain.
➤ **Hormones:** Changes in the body's balance of hormones may be involved in causing or triggering depression. Hormone changes can result with pregnancy and during the weeks or months after delivery (postpartum) and from thyroid problems, menopause or a number of other conditions.
➤ **Inherited traits:** Depression is more common in people whose blood relatives also have this condition. Researchers are trying to find genes that may be involved in causing depression.

Complications

Depression is a serious disorder that can take a terrible toll on the patient and the family.

Examples of complications associated with depression include:

➤ Excess weight or obesity, which can lead to heart disease and diabetes
➤ Family conflicts, relationship difficulties, and work or school problems
➤ Social isolation
➤ Suicidal feelings, suicide attempts or suicide.

SCHIZOPHRENIA

Schizophrenia is a severe mental disorder, affecting 20 million people worldwide.

Symptoms of schizophrenia include:

➤ Hallucinations—hearing or seeing things that do not exist outside of the mind
➤ Delusions—unusual beliefs not based on reality
➤ Muddled thoughts based on hallucinations or delusions
➤ Losing interest in everyday activities
➤ Not caring about your personal hygiene
➤ Wanting to avoid people, including friends

Causes

1. **Genetics:** One of the most significant risk factors for schizophrenia may be genes. This disorder tends to run in families. A person is likely to suffer from schizophrenia if a parent, sibling, or other close relative has suffered from this condition. Other factors, such as stressors, may be needed to "trigger" (listed below) the disorder in people who are at a higher risk.
2. **Brain development:** Studies of people with schizophrenia have shown there are subtle differences in the structure of their brains. These changes are not seen in everyone with schizophrenia and can occur in people who do not have a mental illness. But they suggest schizophrenia may partly be a disorder of the brain.
3. **Chemical changes in the brain:** There is a connection between neurotransmitters and schizophrenia because drugs that alter the levels of neurotransmitters in the brain are known to relieve some of the symptoms of schizophrenia. Research suggests schizophrenia may be caused by a change in the level of 2 neuro-transmitters: Dopamine and serotonin. Some studies indicate an imbalance between the 2 may be the basis of the problem.
4. **Stress:** The main psychological triggers of schizophrenia are stressful life events, such as:
   ➤ Bereavement
   ➤ Losing job
   ➤ Divorce
   ➤ Physical, sexual or emotional abuse

These kinds of experiences, although stressful, do not cause schizophrenia. However, they can trigger its development in someone already vulnerable to it.

Complications

Schizophrenia can be a dangerous disease if it is not treated properly. It can cause complications in many areas of life. Physical problems can occur if the symptoms of schizophrenia are not well controlled. People with schizophrenia are at higher risk for complications such as depression or suicide. They may engage in self-destructive behaviors. People with schizophrenia may get involved in violent crime, either as the victim or as the person committing the crime.

DEMENTIA

Worldwide, approximately 50 million people have dementia. Dementia is usually of a chronic or progressive nature in which there is deterioration in cognitive function (i.e. the ability to process thought) beyond what might be expected from normal ageing. It affects memory, thinking, orientation, comprehension, calculation, learning capacity, language, and judgement. The impairment in cognitive function is commonly accompanied, and occasionally preceded, by deterioration in emotional control, social behavior, or motivation. In later stages of dementia, the patient becomes totally dependent on relatives for all the daily tasks. Dementia is caused by a variety of diseases and injuries that affect the brain, such as Alzheimer's disease or stroke.

Symptoms

Dementia symptoms vary depending on the cause, but common signs and symptoms include:

1. **Cognitive changes**
   - Memory loss, which is usually noticed by a spouse or someone else
   - Difficulty communicating or finding words
   - Difficulty with visual and spatial abilities, such as getting lost while driving
   - Difficulty reasoning or problem-solving
   - Difficulty with planning and organizing
   - Difficulty with coordination and motor functions
   - Confusion and disorientation
2. **Psychological changes**
   - Personality changes
   - Depression
   - Anxiety
   - Inappropriate behavior
   - Paranoia
   - Agitation
   - Hallucinations

Causes

Alzheimer's disease accounts for 60 to 80 percent of cases of dementia. *Vascular dementia,* is the second most common cause of dementia. Dementia is often incorrectly referred to as "senility" or "senile dementia," which reflects the formerly widespread but incorrect belief that serious mental decline is a normal part of aging.

The two types of dementia are associated with particular types of brain cell damage in particular regions of the brain. For example, in Alzheimer's disease, the brain cells of the brain region called the hippocampus are first to be damaged. Hippocampus region is the center of learning and memory in the brain, That is why memory loss is often one of the earliest symptoms of Alzheimer's disease.

Risk Factors for Alzheimer's Dementia

- **Age.** Advancing age is the greatest risk factor for developing Alzheimer's disease. The majority of people diagnosed with Alzheimer's disease are 65 or older.

Although far less common, younger-onset Alzheimer's (also known as early-onset Alzheimer's) affects people younger than 65.

➤ **Family members with Alzheimer's.** A person is more likely to suffer from Alzheimer's disease if a parent or sibling suffered from the disease.

➤ **Genetics.** Genes are estimated to play a role in as many as one-quarter of Alzheimer's cases.

➤ **Cardiovascular disease.** Factors that cause cardiovascular disease also may be linked to a higher risk of developing Alzheimer's and other dementias. Such factors include smoking, obesity, diabetes, and high cholesterol and high blood pressure in midlife.

➤ **Education and Alzheimer's.** Studies have linked fewer years of formal education with an increased risk of Alzheimer's and other dementias.

➤ **Traumatic brain injury.** The risk of Alzheimer's disease and other dementias increases after a moderate or severe traumatic brain injury, such as a blow to the head or injury of the skull that causes amnesia or loss of consciousness for more than 30 minutes.

VASCULAR DEMENTIA

Vascular dementia is the second most common cause of dementia, after Alzheimer's. Common conditions that may lead to vascular dementia include:

➤ **Stroke:** Strokes that block a brain artery usually cause a range of symptoms that may include vascular dementia. But some strokes don't cause any noticeable symptoms. These silent strokes still increase dementia risk. With both silent and apparent strokes, the risk of vascular dementia increases with the number of strokes that occur over time.

➤ **Narrowed or chronically damaged brain blood vessels:** Conditions that narrow or inflict long-term damage on your brain blood vessels also can lead to vascular dementia.

Symptoms of vascular dementia are similar to Alzheimer's disease, although memory loss may not be as apparent in the early stages. Symptoms can sometimes develop suddenly and quickly get worse, but they can also develop gradually over many months or years.

Specific symptoms can include:

➤ *Stroke-like symptoms:* Including muscle weakness or temporary paralysis on one side of the body.

➤ *Movement problems:* Difficulty walking or a change in the way a person walks

Risk Factors

In general, the risk factors for vascular dementia are the same as those for heart disease and stroke.

➤ Increasing age. Your risk of vascular dementia rises as you grow older. The disorder is rare before age 65, and the risk rises substantially by your 90s.

➤ History of heart attack, strokes or ministrokes

➤ Atherosclerosis

➤ High cholesterol

➤ High blood pressure

➤ Diabetes

➤ Smoking

➤ Obesity

CHAPTER

9

Disorders of Gastrointestinal System

PEPTIC ULCER

Peptic ulcer disease presents as duodenal ulcer or gastric ulcer (Fig. 9.1). During the last few decades, the incidence of peptic ulcer disease has decreased in India. In one study, prevalence of duodenal ulcer was 12% in 1988, but it declined to 3 % in 2008. During the same period, gastric ulcer prevalence declined from 4.5% to 2.7%.

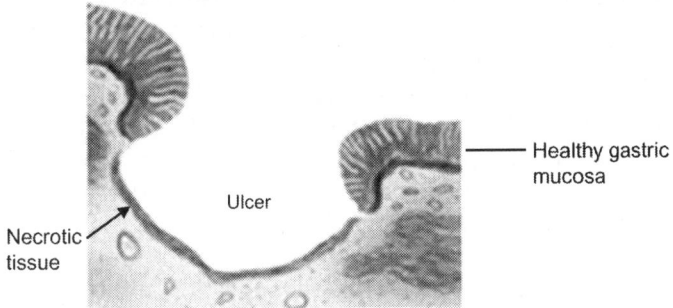

Fig. 9.1: Gastric ulcer

Symptoms

➢ Burning stomach pain. The most common symptoms of a duodenal ulcer are waking at night with upper abdominal pain that improves with eating. With a gastric ulcer, the pain may worsen with eating. The pain is often described as a burning or dull ache.
➢ Feeling of fullness, bloating or belching
➢ Fatty food intolerance
➢ Heart burn
➢ Nausea

Causes of Peptic Ulcer

➢ *H. pylori* infection
➢ NSAIDs

109

➢ Alcohol
➢ Cigarette smoking
➢ Psychogenic stress

Pathogenesis

It is a physiological marvel that gastric juice can easily digest the swallowed pieces of meat but normally, it has no corrosive action on the gastric mucosa itself. Several factors seem to be involved in the protection of gastric mucosa from autodigestion. These factors, collectively known as **gastric mucosal barrier,** include:

a. **Mucus** secreted by surface epithelial cells and mucus neck glands which forms a water insoluble visco-elastic gel with poor diffusion coefficient for H^+.

b. **Bicarbonate** secreted by surface epithelial cells into the boundary zone between the epithelial cells and the mucus layer. The secretion of mucus and bicarbonate is believed to be mediated through prostaglandins.

c. **Tight junctions** between the adjacent cells of gastric surface epithelium.

d. **Rapid turnover** of surface epithelial cells, and rich blood supply.

e. **Prostaglandins.** Endogenous prostaglandins stimulate secretion of gastric mucus as well as gastric and duodenal mucosal bicarbonate. Prostaglandins also participate in the maintenance of gastric mucosal blood flow and integrity of mucosal barrier and promote epithelial cell renewal in response to mucosal injury.

Under normal conditions, a physiologic balance exists between peptic acid secretion and gastro-duodenal mucosal defence. Mucosal injury may lead to peptic ulcer when the balance between the aggressive factors and the defensive mechanisms is disrupted. Aggressive factors, such as *H. pylori*, **NSAIDs, alcohol, cigarette smoking, psychogenic stress** can alter the mucosal defence and allow back diffusion of hydrogen ions and subsequent epithelial cell injury.

Mechanisms of injury differ distinctly between duodenal and gastric ulcers. Duodenal ulcer is essentially a *H. pylori*-related disease and is caused mainly by an increase in acid and pepsin load, and gastric metaplasia in the duodenal cap. Gastric ulcer is most commonly associated with NSAID ingestion, although *H. pylori* infection might also be present. Chronic, superficial and atrophic gastritis predominate in patients with gastric ulcers, when even normal acid levels can be associated with mucosal ulceration.

1. ROLE OF *Helicobacter Pylori*

Helicobacter pylori is a bacillus responsible for one of the most common infections found in humans worldwide. *H. pylori* inhabit the mucus adjacent to the gastric mucosa. *Helicobacter pylori* bacteria colonize the stomach and induce chronic gastritis. *H. pylori* is able to survive the highly acidic environment of the stomach because it protects itself by release of an enzyme urease, that splits blood urea and produces ammonia. The type of ulcer that develops depends on the location of chronic gastritis, which occurs at the site of *H. pylori* colonization.

In those with duodenal ulcer, *H. pylori* colonizes the antrum. The inflammatory response to the bacteria causes destruction of somatostatin-producing D cells in the pylorus. Consequently, the G cells in the antrum secrete more of the hormone gastrin, which travels through the bloodstream to the fundus and body of the stomach. Gastrin stimulates the parietal cells to secrete more acid into the stomach lumen. Chronically increased gastrin levels eventually cause the number of parietal cells to also increase, further escalating the amount of acid secreted. The increased acid load damages the duodenum, and ulceration may eventually result.

In contrast, in gastric ulcers, H. pylori colonize the corpus of the stomach, where the acid-secreting parietal cells are located. However, chronic inflammation induced by the bacteria leads to reduction of acid production, and eventually atrophy of the stomach lining. Gastric atrophy may lead to gastric ulcer and increases the risk for stomach cancer.

2. NON-STEROIDAL ANTI-INFLAMMATORY DRUGS

Non-steroidal anti-inflammatory drugs (NSAIDs) including low-dose aspirin are some of the most commonly used medicines. They are associated with gastrointestinal mucosal injury. Endoscopic studies have shown a prevalence rate of 14–25% of gastric and duodenal ulcers in NSAID users, NSAID acts as anti-inflammatory agents by inhibition of prostaglandin (PG) synthesis. As discussed earlier, prostaglandins are important component of gastric mucosal barrier. Inhibition of PG synthesis breaks gastric mucosal barrier leading to peptic ulcers.

3. SMOKING

Cigarette smoking appears to be a risk factor for the development, maintenance, and recurrence of peptic ulcer disease. Smokers are about two times as likely to develop ulcer disease as non-smokers. Smoking predisposes to peptic ulcer by (i) acceleration of gastric emptying of liquids, (ii) promotion of duodeno-gastric reflux, (iii) reduction in mucosal blood flow, and (iv) inhibition of mucosal prostaglandin production. Cigarette smoking not only causes ulcer formation, but also increases the risk of ulcer complications such as ulcer bleeding, stomach obstruction and perforation. Since cessation of smoking is associated with the prompt recovery of the respective functions, smokers will benefit immediately by stopping or reducing cigarette consumption. Cigarette smoking is also a leading cause of failure of medicinal treatment of peptic ulcer.

4. ROLE OF STRESS

The development of acute gastric ulcers as a result of severe stress after major surgery or extensive burns is well known. Reduced gastric blood flow coupled with raised plasma cortisol levels seem to be primarily responsible for such ulcers.

Till 1980s, psychological stress was considered the chief cause of duodenal ulcer. The high stung type "A" individuals were considered special candidates for the development of duodenal ulcer. In 1990s, after the discovery of H. pylori, it began to be believed that psychogenic factors play no role in the development of chronic peptic ulcer disease. Over the years, it is now being appreciated that psychogenic stress acts as a co-factor with H. pylori in the production of hyperacidity leading to duodenal ulcer.

Risk Factors

➢ Alcohol   ➢ Spicy food

Alone, these factors do not cause ulcers, but they can make them worse and more difficult to heal.

Complications

Left untreated, peptic ulcers can result in serious complications:

➢ **Internal bleeding.** Bleeding can occur as slow blood loss that leads to anemia or as severe blood loss that may require hospitalization or a blood transfusion. Severe blood loss may cause black or bloody vomit or black or bloody stools.

➢ **Infection.** Peptic ulcers can perforate the wall of stomach putting at risk of serious infection called peritonitis.

➢ Obstruction to the passage of food (Fig. 9.2).

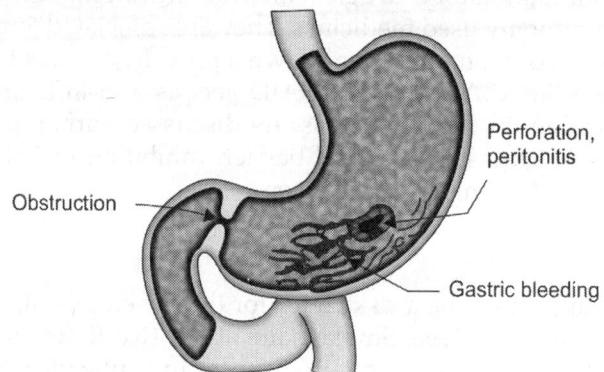

Fig. 9.2: Complications of peptic ulcer

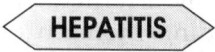

Hepatitis is an inflammation of the liver. The condition can be self-limiting or can progress to fibrosis (scarring), cirrhosis or liver cancer. Hepatitis viruses are the most common cause of hepatitis in the world but other infections, toxic substances (e.g. alcohol, certain drugs), and autoimmune diseases can also cause hepatitis.

VIRAL HEPATITIS

Viral hepatitis is one of the major public health concerns around the world. Every year 1.4 million people die from viral hepatitis-related cirrhosis and liver cancer. Viral hepatitis is a cause for major health care burden in India as well.

There are 5 main hepatitis viruses, referred to as types A, B, C, D and E. Viral hepatitis A, B and E is an acute disorder. Types B and C lead to chronic hepatitis in hundreds of millions of people and, together, are the most common cause of liver cirrhosis and cancer.

Hepatitis A virus (HAV) is present in the faeces of infected persons and is most often transmitted through consumption of contaminated water or food.

Most people in areas of the world with poor sanitation have been infected with this virus.

Hepatitis B virus (HBV) is transmitted through exposure to infective blood, semen, and other body fluids. Transmission occurs through transfusions of HBV-contaminated blood and blood products, contaminated injections during medical procedures, and through injection drug use. HBV also poses a risk to healthcare workers who sustain accidental needle stick injuries while caring for infected-HBV patients.

Hepatitis C virus (HCV) is mostly transmitted through exposure to infective blood. This may happen through transfusions of HCV-contaminated blood and blood products, contaminated injections during medical procedures, and through injection drug use. Sexual transmission is also possible, but is much less common.

Hepatitis D virus (HDV) infections occur only in those who are infected with HBV. The dual infection of HDV and HBV can result in a more serious disease and worse outcome.

Hepatitis E virus (HEV) is mostly transmitted through consumption of contaminated water or food. HEV is a common cause of hepatitis outbreaks in developing parts of the world and is increasingly recognized as an important cause of disease in developed countries.

Symptoms and Signs of Hepatitis A

➢ Fatigue
➢ Sudden nausea and vomiting
➢ Abdominal pain or discomfort, especially on the upper right side beneath lower ribs (site of liver)
➢ Clay-colored stools
➢ Loss of appetite
➢ Low-grade fever
➢ Jaundice
➢ Dark urine
➢ Joint pain
➢ Intense itching

Pathology of Acute Hepatitis (Fig. 9.3)

The characteristic histopathological features of acute hepatitis include:
➢ Ballooning degeneration
➢ Spotty necrosis
➢ Predominantly sinusoidal and lobular mononuclear cell infiltrate
➢ Kupffer cell hyperplasia
➢ Scattered apoptotic bodies
➢ Hepatocellular regeneration

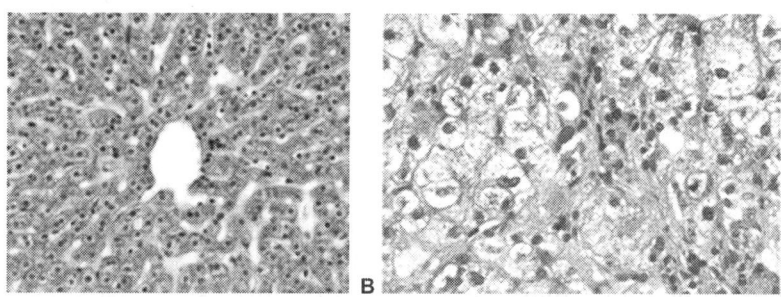

Fig. 9.3: Histology liver. (A) Normal; (B) acute viral hepatitis

Complication of Acute Hepatitis

➢ Hepatic failure

Complications of Chronic Hepatitis

➢ Hepatic failure
➢ Liver cirrhosis
➢ Hepatic cancer

<JAUNDICE>

Jaundice is a yellow discoloration of the skin, mucous membranes, and the whites of the eyes caused by increased amounts of bilirubin in the blood. Serum bilirubin level is normally below 1.0 mg/dL, and levels over 2–3 mg/dL typically results in jaundice.

▌BILIRUBIN METABOLISM (FIG. 9.4)

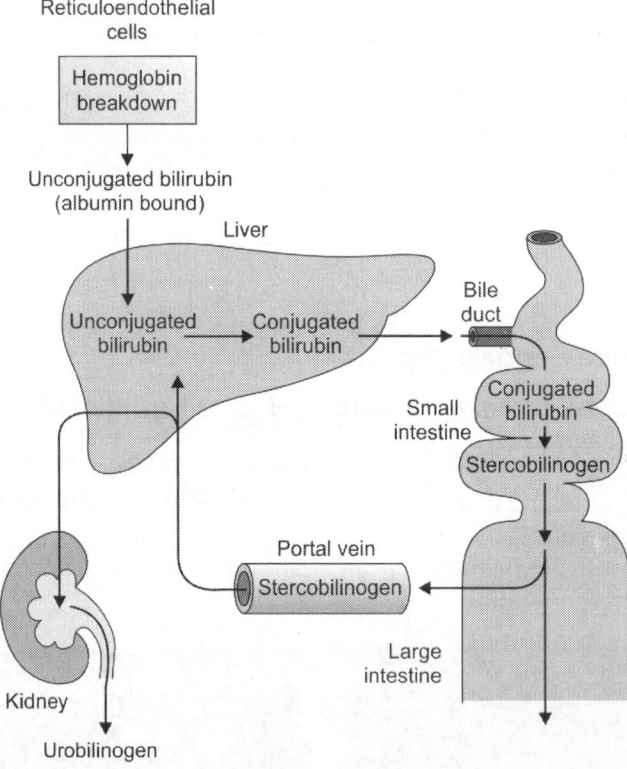

Fig. 9.4: Bilirubin metabolism

Destruction of senescent red blood cells in the tissue macrophages (in spleen, liver, bone marrow, etc.) results in catabolism of haemoglobin to haeme (and globin) and subsequently to bilirubin. Bilirubin released from the tissue macrophages is called unconjugated bilirubin. It a lipid soluble pigment transported in blood tightly bound to albumin. In the liver, the hepatocytes take up unconjugated bilirubin from the blood, convert it into water-soluble compounds called conjugated bilirubin (bilirubin mono- and di-glucuronide), and excrete it into bile canaliculi. Bile duct excretes conjugated bilirubin into small intestine.

Conjugated bilirubin cannot be absorbed in the intestines. In the large gut, bacterial degradation converts it to stercobilinogen (= urobilinogen), a water soluble colourless product. Some of the urobilinogen is absorbed into the portal blood to reach the systemic circulation. Being water soluble, it is excreted into the urine by the kidneys. The remaining stercobilinogen is excreted in the faeces. On exposure to air, stercobilinogen is oxidized to stercobilin which gives brown color to the faeces.

In obstructive jaundice, since bilirubin does not reach the intestines, stercobilinogen and urobilinogen excretion in the faeces and urine is very low. That accounts for the pale chalky-color of the stools of such patients.

Conjugated bilirubin is water-soluble; if present in the blood, it is excreted by the kidneys into the urine (bilirubinuria). Bilirubin imparts dark brown color to the urine, an important clinical sign of conjugated hyperbilirubinemias (hepatic and post-hepatic jaundice). Classification of jaundice based on the pathophysiology of bilirubin metabolism is given below:

Jaundice type	Definition
Pre-hepatic/ haemolytic	The pathology is occurring prior to the liver in bilirubin metabolism. It can be due to either: A. Increased haemolysis due to intrinsic (congenital) defects in red blood cells B. Extrinsic causes of increased haemolysis.
Hepatic/hepato-cellular	The pathology is located within the liver due to disease of parenchymal cells of liver.
Post-hepatic	The pathology is located after the conjugation of bilirubin in the liver, due to obstruction in biliary passage.

PRE-HEPATIC JAUNDICE

Pre-hepatic jaundice is caused by an increased rate of haemolysis due to a congenital (sickle cell anemia, spherocytosis, thalassemia) or an acquired defect in the structure of red cells. (*See* Chapter 6, hemolytic anemia.) The increased breakdown of red blood cells leads to an increase in the production of unconjugated bilirubin. Presence of excess of unconjugated bilirubin in blood causes its deposition into various tissues causing jaundice. Increased production of unconjugated bilirubin leads to increased production and increased excretion of stercobilinogen and urobilinogen in stools and urine respectively. Bilirubin is not found in the urine because unconjugated bilirubin is not water-soluble.

Laboratory findings include:
➤ Urine: Excess of urobilinogen, absent bilirubin.
➤ Serum: Increased unconjugated bilirubin.

HEPATIC JAUNDICE

Hepatocellular (hepatic) jaundice results from an acute or chronic injury to hepatocytes (viral hepatitis, cirrhosis, alcoholic liver disease). Cell necrosis reduces the liver's ability to take up, conjugate and excrete bilirubin. Therefore, level of both unconjugated and conjugated type of bilirubin rises in the blood. The conjugated type of bilirubin, when present in the blood is excreted in the urine.

Laboratory findings include:
➤ *Urine:* Bilirubin present.
➤ Serum contains excess of both conjugated and unconjugated bilirubin.
➤ Elevated levels of certain enzymes in the blood indicative of hepatocellular injury.

POST-HEPATIC JAUNDICE

Post-hepatic jaundice, also called obstructive jaundice, is caused by an interruption to the drainage of bile, containing conjugated bilirubin, in the biliary system. The most common causes are gallstones in the common bile duct, and cancer in the head of the pancreas, through which the bile duct passes. The back pressure on bile causes regurgitation of conjugated bilirubin and bile salts into blood circulation.

In complete obstruction of the bile duct, bile does not reach the intestine, stercobilinogen and urobilinogen are not found in the faeces and urine, restively. Hence faeces have a pale chalky appearance.

Laboratory findings include:
➤ Urine: Bilirubin present, urobilinogen absent
➤ Serum contains excess of conjugated bilirubin.

ALCOHOL LIVER DISEASE

Alcohol consumption is on the rise in India. Between 2010 and 2017, alcohol consumption in India increased by 38 per cent. In some parts of India, the prevalence of current alcohol use varies between 33% and 50%, with a higher prevalence among the lesser educated and the poor. In India, 15 people die every day from the effects of drinking alcohol.

Chronic heavy drinking may lead to:
➤ Alcoholic fatty liver
➤ Alcoholic hepatitis
➤ Alcoholic cirrhosis (Laënnec's cirrhosis) (Fig. 9.5)

Between 10 and 20 percent of heavy drinkers will develop cirrhosis. Alcohol liver disease starts as alcoholic fatty liver. It then progress to alcoholic hepatitis, and then to alcoholic cirrhosis. Alcoholic liver cirrhosis is the most advanced form of liver disease that is related to drinking alcohol. Liver cirrhosis ends up as liver failure.

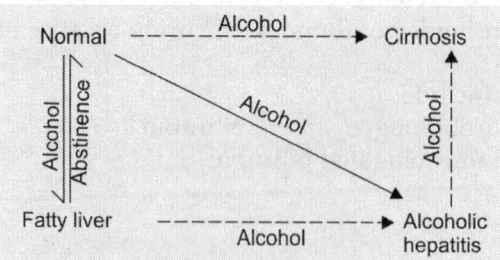

Fig. 9.5: Possible pathways of liver cirrhosis in alcoholics

Symptoms and Signs

a. Alcoholic fatty liver

➤ Usually no symptoms
➤ Discomfort in right upper abdomen (liver region)
➤ Fatigue

b. Alcoholic hepatitis

➤ Jaundice
➤ Fatigue
➤ Loss of appetite
➤ Low grade fever

➤ Nausea
➤ Vomiting
➤ Tenderness in right upper abdomen

c. Alcoholic cirrhosis

➤ Fatigue
➤ Loss of appetite
➤ Nausea
➤ Ankles edema

➤ Weight loss
➤ Jaundice
➤ Ascites

PATHOGENESIS OF ALCOHOL LIVER DISEASE

In alcoholic liver disease, the total amount and duration of ethanol ingested rather than the type of alcoholic drink ingested determines the results. For example, 360 ml of beer (5% alcohol) and 45 ml of whisky contain the same amount of ethanol. Women appear to develop alcohol-induced liver injury at lesser levels of consumption than men. Malnutrition seems to augment the detrimental effects of alcohol. The cause of malnutrition in alcoholics is not merely economic. Even when economic problem is not present, alcoholism tends to produce malnutrition. In chronic alcoholics, alcohol itself may provide over 50% of total caloric requirements, which otherwise would have been provided by food containing proteins, vitamins and minerals.

Liver is the main site of alcohol metabolism. In the hepatocytes, alcohol is first oxidized to acetaldehyde, which is further oxidized to acetate (Fig. 9.6). Both of these reactions increase the concentration of NADH which inhibits the operation of citric

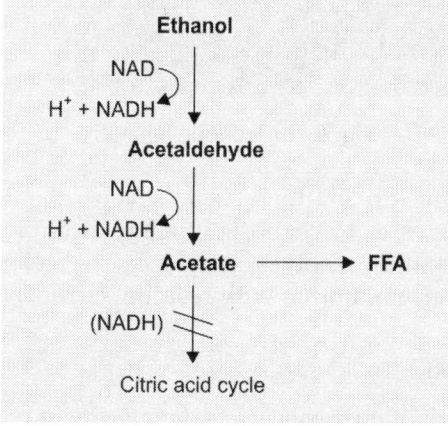

Fig. 9.6: Biochemical basis of alcohol-induced hepatic injury

acid cycle. Therefore, rather than undergoing further oxidation to CO_2 and water, acetate is diverted to fatty acid synthesis.

Alcohol causes inhibition of fatty acid oxidation as well. Excessive concentration of acetaldehyde seems to inhibit biosynthesis and secretion of lipoproteins, the form in which fatty acids can be exported from the liver. Therefore, triglycerides accumulate in the hepatocytes, producing "fatty liver" (Fig. 1.15). Fatty liver may develop in any alcoholic after a bout of heavy drinking, but it is a reversible process. This condition presents clinically as a tender hepatomegaly with many non-specific symptoms such as malaise, weakness, anorexia, nausea, and abdominal discomfort. Elevated levels of hepatic enzymes may be the only laboratory finding. Jaundice is present in 15% of patients admitted to the hospital because of these symptoms of fatty infiltration of the liver. With total abstinence, the condition can return to normal within 2-4 weeks. However, continued alcohol consumption may result in more advanced forms of liver disease, either alcoholic hepatitis or cirrhosis.

ALCOHOLIC HEPATITIS

Some 10–15% of chronic alcoholics develop alcoholic hepatitis. Alcoholic hepatitis is characterized by hepatocyte ballooning, hepatocyte necrosis and polymorphonuclear infiltration (Fig. 9.7). Deposition of collagen fibers around the central vein and in peri-sinusoidal area sets the stage for progression to cirrhosis. Cardinal sign of alcoholic hepatitis is rapid onset of jaundice. Other common features include fever and ascites.

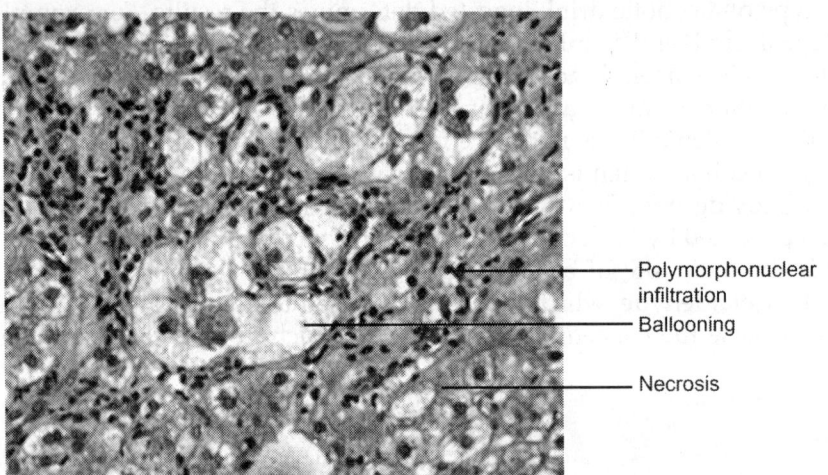

Fig. 9.7: Alcoholic hepatitis

Encephalopathy may develop in those with severe hepatitis. Alcoholic hepatitis usually persists and progresses to cirrhosis if heavy alcohol use continues. If alcohol use ceases, alcoholic hepatitis resolves slowly over weeks to months, sometimes without permanent sequelae but often with residual cirrhosis.

ALCOHOLIC CIRRHOSIS

The pathological hallmark of cirrhosis is the development of scar tissue that replaces normal hepatic parenchyma, blocking the portal flow of blood through the organ and disturbing normal function. The fibrous tissue bands (septa) separate hepatocyte nodules; which eventually distort the entire liver architecture (Fig. 9.8), and obstruct the normal hepatic blood flow leading to portal hypertension. Alcoholic liver cirrhosis is the most advanced form of liver disease that is related to drinking alcohol. Portal hypertension is responsible for most severe complications of cirrhosis such as edema feet, ascites and bleeding from esophageal varices.

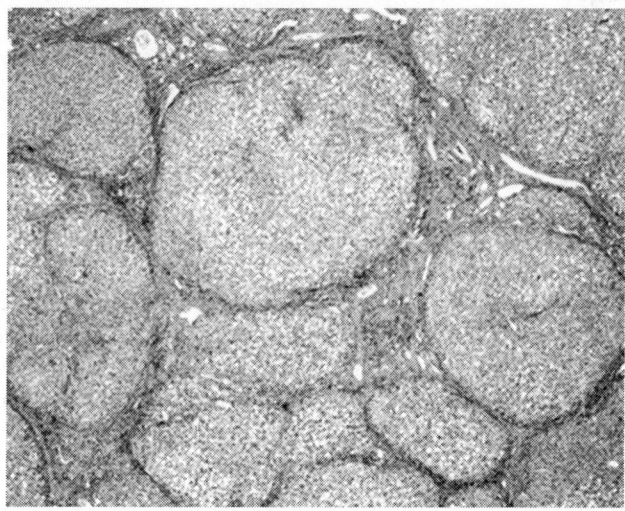

Fig. 9.8: Liver cirrhosis

Complications of Liver Cirrhosis

➤ Ascites
➤ Edema feet
➤ Bacterial peritonitis

➤ Bleeding from esophageal varices
➤ Hepatic encephalopathy (hepatic coma)
➤ Liver cancer

INFLAMMATORY BOWEL DISEASE

Inflammatory bowel disease (IBD) is an umbrella term used to describe disorders that involve chronic inflammation of your digestive tract. Types of IBD include:

1. ULCERATIVE COLITIS

In ulcerative colitis, inflammation begins in the rectum and extends proximally in an uninterrupted fashion to the proximal colon, eventually involving the entire length of the large intestine. The small intestine is never involved. The rectum is always involved in ulcerative colitis, and no "skip areas" (i.e. normal areas of the bowel interspersed with diseased areas) are present. Ulcerative colitis primarily involves the mucosa and the submucosa, with formation of crypt abscesses and mucosal.

2. CROHN'S DISEASE

In Crohn's disease, the most common location is the ileocecal region, followed by the terminal ileum Diseased segments frequently are separated by intervening normal bowel, leading to the term "skip areas." Inflammation can be transmural (extending through the entire depth of intestinal wall), often extending through to the serosa, resulting in sinus tracts or fistula formation.

Signs and symptoms that are common to both Crohn's disease and ulcerative colitis include:
> ➤ Diarrhea
> ➤ Fever and fatigue
> ➤ Abdominal pain and cramping
> ➤ Blood in your stool
> ➤ Reduced appetite
> ➤ Unintended weight loss

Cause

The exact cause of inflammatory bowel disease remains unknown. One possible cause is an immune system malfunction.
> ➤ **Age.** Most people who develop IBD are diagnosed before they are 30 years old.
> ➤ **Family history.** You are at higher risk if you have a close relative—such as a parent, sibling or child—with the disease.
> ➤ **Cigarette smoking.** Cigarette smoking is the most important controllable risk factor for developing Crohn's disease.
> ➤ **Nonsteroidal anti-inflammatory medications.** These medications may increase the risk of developing IBD or worsen disease in people who have IBD.

Complications

> ➤ **Colon cancer.** Having IBD increases your risk of colon cancer. General colon cancer screening guidelines for people without IBD call for a colonoscopy every 10 years beginning at age 50. Ask your doctor whether you need to have this test done sooner and more frequently.
> ➤ **Skin, eye and joint inflammation.** Certain disorders, including arthritis, skin lesions and eye inflammation (uveitis), may occur during IBD flare-ups.
> ➤ **Bowel obstruction.** Crohn's disease affects the full thickness of the intestinal wall. Over time, parts of the bowel can thicken and narrow, which may block the flow of digestive contents. You may require surgery to remove the diseased portion of your bowel.
> ➤ **Malnutrition.** Diarrhea, abdominal pain and cramping may make it difficult for you to eat or for your intestine to absorb enough nutrients to keep you nourished. It is also common to develop anemia due to low iron or vitamin B_{12} caused by the disease.
> ➤ **Ulcers.** Chronic inflammation can lead to open sores (ulcers) anywhere in your digestive tract, including your mouth and anus, and in the genital area (perineum).

Disorders of Bones and Joints

CHAPTER

10

RHEUMATOID ARTHRITIS

Rheumatoid arthritis (RA) is characterized by inflammation and swelling of the synovial membrane of the joint, with subsequent destruction of articular structures. RA affects about 1% of Indian population.

Aetiology

Rheumatoid arthritis is an autoimmune disorder of the synovial joints and other organs of the body.

Symptoms

Signs and symptoms of rheumatoid arthritis may include:
➢ Tender, warm, swollen joints
➢ Joint stiffness that is usually worse in the mornings
➢ Fatigue
➢ Fever
➢ Loss of appetite

Early rheumatoid arthritis tends to affect smaller joints first—particularly the joints that attach fingers to the hands and toes to the feet. As the disease progresses, symptoms often spread to the wrists, knees, ankles, elbows, hips and shoulders. In most cases, symptoms occur in the same joints on both sides of the body. Loss of movement and erosion of the joint surface lead to deformity and loss of function of the joint (Fig. 10.1). About 40 percent of the people who have rheumatoid arthritis also experience signs and symptoms in other body systems, cardiovascular system in particular.

PATHOPHYSIOLOGY

RA typically manifests with signs of inflammation of the synovial membrane. The affected joint is swollen, warm, painful and stiff, particularly early in the morning on waking. The resulting inflammation thickens the synovial membrane, which can eventually destroy the cartilage and bone within the joint (Fig. 10.2).

As the pathology progresses, the inflammatory activity leads to tendon damage as well as erosion and destruction of the joint surface, which impairs range of movement

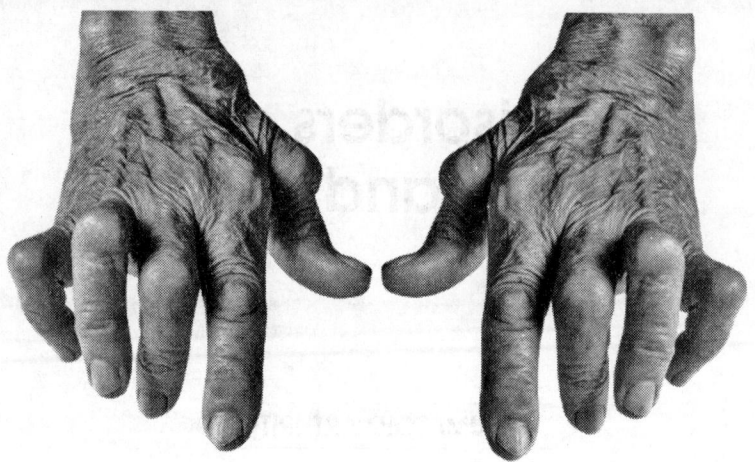

Fig. 10.1: Deformed fingers in a patient with rheumatoid arthritis

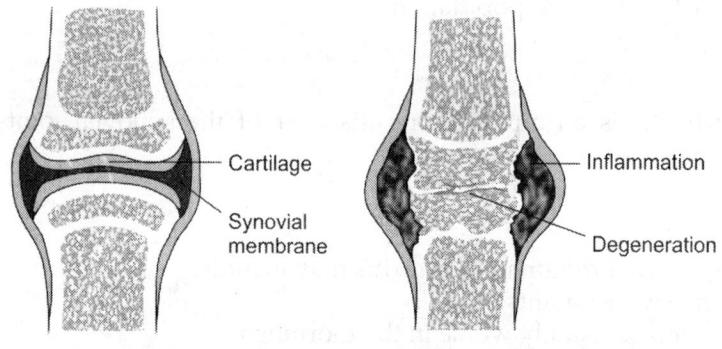

Fig. 10.2: Condition of synovial joint in rheumatoid arthritis

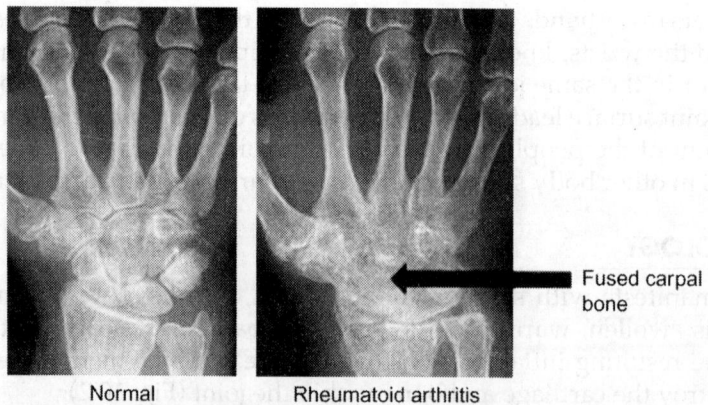

Fig. 10.3: Fused bones of the wrist in rheumatoid arthritis

and leads to deformity. Gradually, the joint loses its shape and alignment. Destruction and fusion of bones of the wrist (carpal bones) is commonly observed (Fig. 10.3). The skin, bones, and muscles adjacent to the joints atrophy from disuse and destruction.

Risk Factors

➢ **Sex.** Women are more likely than men to develop rheumatoid arthritis.
➢ **Age.** Rheumatoid arthritis can occur at any age, but it most commonly begins in middle age.
➢ **Family history.** The risk of developing RA is greater, if there is family history of the disease.
➢ **Smoking.** Cigarette smoking increases risk of developing rheumatoid arthritis. Moreover, smoking also appears to be associated with greater disease severity.

Complications

➢ Osteoporosis, partly because of drugs used in the treatment of the disorder.
➢ Coronary artery disease   ➢ Eye inflammation
➢ Stroke   ➢ Anemia
➢ Lung fibrosis   ➢ Depression

OSTEOARTHRITIS

Osteoarthritis is the most common chronic musculoskeletal disorder. Epidemiological studies estimate that it affects about 15% of the world population. In contrast to the inflammatory cause of rheumatoid arthritis, osteoarthritis is a degenerative disease (Fig. 10.4). It occurs when the protective cartilage that cushions the ends of your bones wears down over time. The **most common joints affected** by osteoarthritis are the **small joints** of the hands and feet, the **hip joint,** and the **knee joint**.

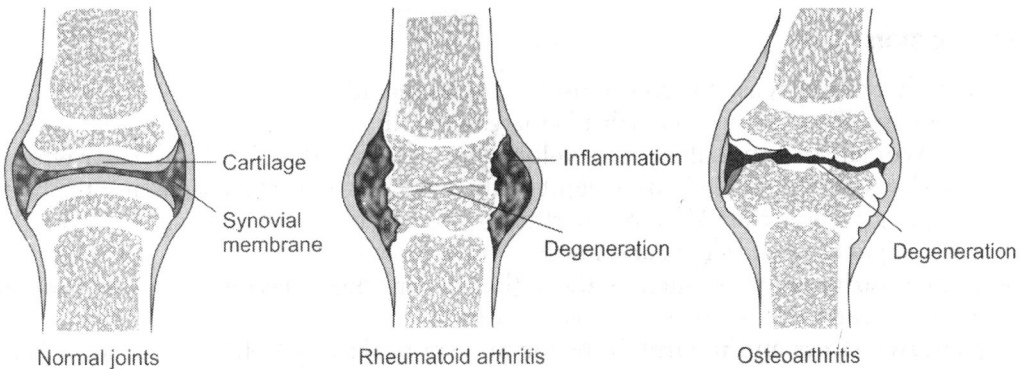

Fig. 10.4: Difference between rheumatoid arthritis and osteoarthritis

Symptoms

➢ Pain or aching in the joint during activity, after long activity or at the end of the day.
➢ Joint stiffness usually occurs first thing in the morning or after resting.
➢ Limited range of motion that may go away after movement.

➢ Clicking or cracking sound when a joint bends.
➢ Swelling around a joint.
➢ Muscle weakness around the joint.
➢ Joint instability or buckling (knee gives out).

Aetiology

Osteoarthritis occurs when the cartilage that cushions the ends of bones in the joints gradually deteriorates. Cartilage is a firm, slippery tissue that enables nearly frictionless joint motion. Eventually, if the cartilage wears down completely, bone will rub on bone.

Pathogenesis

Earlier, osteoarthritis has been considered to be a disease involving wear and tear of articular cartilage. Remnants of degenerated cartilage are found in the joint (Fig. 10.5). Recent research has indicated that the condition involves the entire joint. The loss of articular cartilage is the primary change, but a combination of cellular changes and biomechanical stresses causes several secondary changes, including subchondral bone remodelling, the formation of new bone at the joint margins called osteophytes and degenerative changes in joint capsule, ligaments and periarticular muscles.

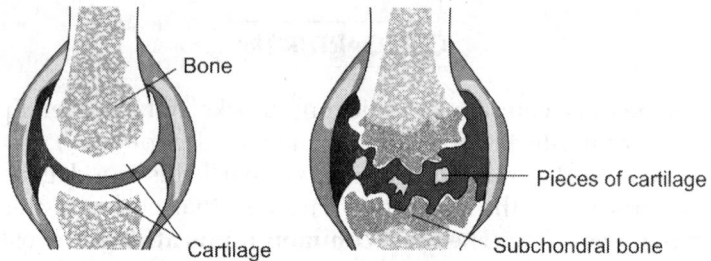

Bone

Pieces of cartilage

Cartilage

Subchondral bone

Fig. 10.5: Degeneration of articular cartilage and bone in osteoarthritis

Risk Factors

Factors that can increase the risk of osteoarthritis include:
➢ **Older age.** The risk of osteoarthritis increases with age.
➢ **Sex.** Women are more likely to develop osteoarthritis, though it is not clear why.
➢ **Obesity.** Carrying extra body weight contributes to osteoarthritis. Greater the body weight, greater is the risk of osteoarthritis. Increased weight adds stress to weight-bearing joints, such as hips and knees.
➢ **Joint injuries.** Injuries, such as those that occur when playing sports or from an accident, can increase the risk of osteoarthritis.
➢ **Repeated stress on the joint.** If the job or a sport places repetitive stress on a joint, that joint might eventually develop osteoarthritis.
➢ **Genetics.** Some people inherit a tendency to develop osteoarthritis.

Complications

➢ Osteoarthritis is a degenerative disease that worsens over time, often resulting in chronic pain. Joint pain and stiffness can become severe enough to make daily tasks difficult.

➢ Depression and sleep disturbances can result from the pain and disability of osteoarthritis.

◁ OSTEOPOROSIS ▷

Osteoporosis is characterized by reduced bone mass and the disruption of normal bone architecture (Fig. 10.6). The result is fragility of bone that is easily fractured. Osteoporosis occurs in both men and women, but it sets in early and is more severe in women. Around the world, 1 in 3 women and 1 in 5 men aged fifty years and over are at risk of an osteoporotic fracture. As explained below, Indians have lower bone mass as adults and hence are more prone to develop osteoporosis.

Osteoporosis seen in cases with immobilization or hormonal disorders such as Cushing syndrome or thyrotoxicosis is known as *secondary osteoporosis. Senile osteoporosis in men and postmenopausal osteoporosis is far more common.*

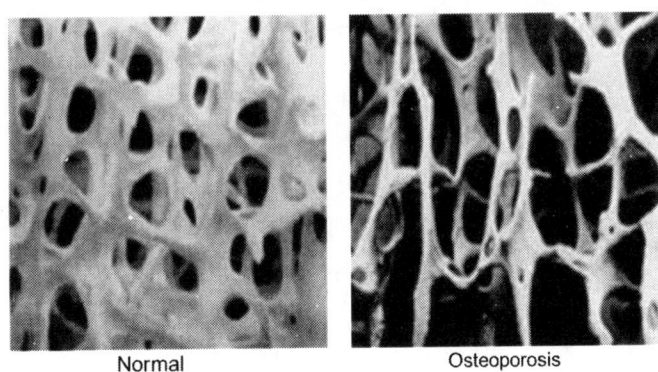

Normal   Osteoporosis

Fig. 10.6: Architecture of bone—normal and in osteoporosis

Symptoms

There typically are no symptoms in the early stages of bone loss. But once bones have been weakened by osteoporosis, signs and symptoms include:
➢ Back pain, caused by a fractured or collapsed vertebra
➢ Loss of height over time
➢ A stooped posture
➢ A bone that breaks much more easily than expected

Hip fractures often are caused by a fall and can result in disability and even an increased risk of death within the first year after the injury.

Aetiology and Risk Factors

The exact cause of **senile/postmenopausal osteoporosis** is not known. However, certain risk factors have been identified:

1. Peak Bone Mass

Peak bone mass has been identified as one of the most important factors in the pathogenesis of osteoporosis. Maximum bone mass is attained in both men and women at around the age of 30 years. A failure to attain optimal bone strength by this point is one factor that contributes to osteoporosis later in life.

Bone is a living tissue. All the time some part of bone is being resorbed and new bone is laid out. This process is known as bone remodelling. After the age of 30 years, the *remodelling process involves slightly greater bone resorption than bone deposition.* Thus, the age-related bone loss gradually sets in. By the age of 60 years in men, and approximately a decade earlier in women, the loss of bone mass becomes significant (Fig. 10.7). Osteoporosis sets in earlier in those with low peak bone mass. The racial difference in peak bone mass is reflected in the incidence of severe osteoporosis. In American population, peak bone mass is significantly greater in blacks than whites. The incidence of fracture femoral neck (severe osteoporosis) is significantly greater in whites than blacks. Indians in general have low peak bone mass. Twin and family studies have shown that *genetic factors play an important role* in regulating bone mineral density and bone turnover.

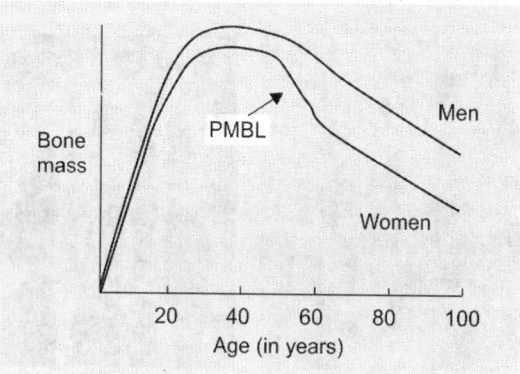

Fig. 10.7: Age and sex related loss of bone mass. (PMBL = postmenopausal bone loss)

2. Gonadal Hormonal Deficiency

Ageing and loss of gonadal function are the 2 most important factors contributing to the development of osteoporosis. Estrogen or testosterone deficiency, regardless of age of occurrence, results in accelerated bone loss. The exact mechanisms of this bone loss is not clear. Whatever the mechanism, ultimately there is an increased bone resorption, which outpaces bone formation. Studies have shown that bone loss in women accelerates rapidly in the first years after menopause.

Blood gonadal hormone levels decline with age both in male and females. However, the postmenopausal precipitous fall in blood estrogen level observed in females does not occur in blood testosterone levels in male; blood testosterone levels in males decline more gradually.

3. Dietary Calcium and Vitamin D

Dietary calcium and vitamin D intake during the first three decades of life is an important factor since it determines the value of peak bone mass.

4. Exercise

At any age, immobilization with decreased weight bearing leads to rapid bone resorption. Physical activity, muscle strength and body weight seem to be important determinants of bone strength. Osteoporotic subjects in general are less muscular and have lower body weight.

5. Excessive Intake of Acids

High acid intake, particularly in the form of high protein diet may contribute to the development of osteoporosis; bone is involved in buffering the acid load. Acidosis may also increase the osteoclastic activity by a direct action.

Complications

Bone fractures, particularly in the spine or hip, are the most serious complications of osteoporosis.

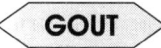

Gout is characterized by sudden, severe attacks of pain, swelling, redness and tenderness in the joints, often the joint at the base of the big toe. In western countries, gout occurs in 3–6% in men and 1–2% in women. In India, prevalence of gout is much less, around 0.1%.

Symptoms and Signs

The signs and symptoms of gout almost always occur suddenly, and often at night. They include:

➤ **Intense joint pain.** Gout usually affects the large joint of the big toe, but it can occur in any joint. Other commonly affected joints include the ankles, knees, elbows, wrists and fingers. The pain is likely to be most severe within the first four to 12 hours after it begins.

➤ **Inflammation and redness.** The affected joint or joints become swollen, tender, warm and red (Fig. 10.8).

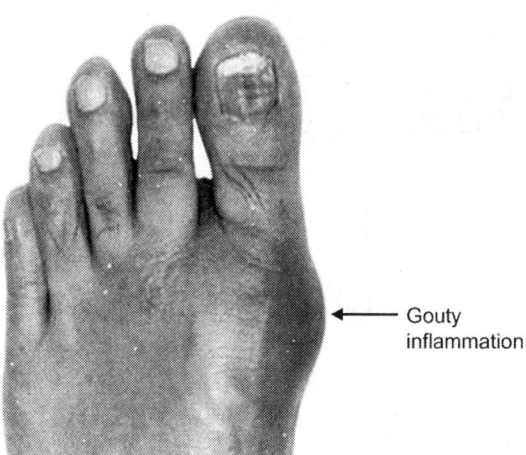

Gouty inflammation

Fig. 10.8: Gout

> ➢ **Lingering discomfort.** After the most severe pain subsides, some joint discomfort may last from a few days to a few weeks. Later attacks are likely to last longer and affect more joints.
> ➢ **Limited range of motion.** As gout progresses, movement in the joint becomes limit.

Causes

Gout occurs when urate crystals accumulate in a joint, causing the inflammation and intense pain. Urate crystals can form when a patient has high serum uric acid level.

Pathogenesis

Uric acid is normally produced in our body in the catabolism of purines. Purines are also found in certain foods, such as organ meats and seafood. Other foods also promote higher levels of uric acid, such as alcoholic beverages, especially beer, and drinks sweetened with fructose. Normally, uric acid remains dissolved in the blood and excreted by the kidneys into the urine. But sometimes serum uric acid rises due to either greater uric acid production in the body, or more often, decreased excretion by the kidneys. When this happens, uric acid can be deposited as sharp, needle-like urate crystals in a joint or surrounding tissue that cause pain, inflammation and swelling (Fig. 10.9).

These crystals initiate the inflammatory process by being engulfed by synovial phagocytic cells leading to release of lysosomal enzymes and production of inflammatory chemokines. The chemotactic factors produced by monocytes and mast cells and the local vasodilatation stimulates neutrophilic chemotaxis. Also, endothelial cells activation further aggravates the inflammatory response and migration of neutrophils. The chemokines attract neutrophils into the synovial tissue and the synovial fluid.

The way to ultimately correct the underlying metabolic problem of hyperuricemia and the crystal deposition is to lower the serum urate level and dissolve the crystal deposits by medicines. This will stop both the acute attacks and the progressive joint damage.

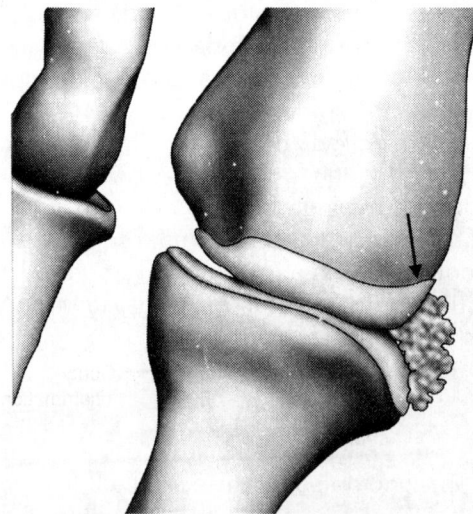

Fig. 10.9: Urate crystals in a joint

Risk Factors

Factors that increase the uric acid level in the body include:

➢ **Diet.** Eating a diet rich in meat and seafood and drinking beverages sweetened with fruit sugar (fructose) increase levels of uric acid. Alcohol consumption, especially of beer, also increases the risk of gout.

➢ **Obesity.** If one is overweight, the body produces more uric acid.

➢ **Medical conditions.** Certain diseases increase the risk of gout. These include hypertension, diabetes, metabolic syndrome, and heart and kidney diseases.

➢ **Certain medications.** The use of thiazide diuretics—commonly used to treat hypertension—and low-dose aspirin also can increase uric acid levels.

➢ **Family history of gout**

➢ **Age and sex.** Gout occurs more often in men, primarily because women tend to have lower uric acid levels. After menopause, however, women's uric acid levels approach those of men. Men are also more likely to develop gout earlier—usually between the ages of 30 and 50, whereas women generally develop signs and symptoms after menopause.

Complications

People with gout can develop more severe conditions, such as:

➢ **Joint destruction.** If left untreated, gout can cause erosion and destruction of a joint.

➢ **Urate tophi.** Untreated gout may cause deposits of urate crystals to form under the skin in nodules called tophi. Tophi can develop in several areas such as your fingers, hands, feet, elbows or Achilles tendons.

➢ **Kidney stones.** Urate crystals may collect in the urinary tract of people with gout, causing kidney stones.

Principles of Cancer

According to Indian Council of Medical Research, more than 1300 Indians die every day due to cancer. Between 2012 and 2014, the mortality rate due to cancer increased by approximately 6%. In India cancer of breast, lung and stomach are more common.

TUMOR

➢ Tumor is a mass of cells which results from an abnormal proliferation of cells.
➢ A tumor can be either **benign** or **malignant (Fig. 11.1).**
➢ **Benign tumor:** A tumor that remains confined to its original location, neither invading surrounding normal tissue nor spreading to distant body sites is known as benign tumor.
➢ **Malignant tumor:** A tumor which is capable of both invading surrounding normal tissue and spreading (metastasis) throughout the body via the circulatory or lymphatic systems is known as malignant tumor. Only malignant tumors are referred to as cancer.

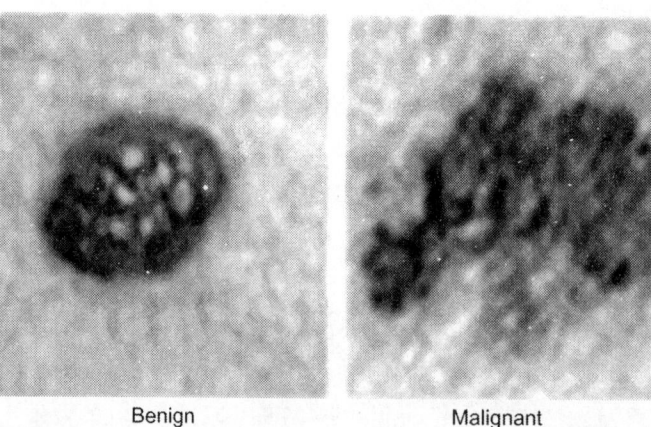

Benign   Malignant

Fig. 11.1: Gross appearance of a benign and malignant tumor

The differences between benign and malignant tumors are described in Table 11.1.

Table 11.1	Differences between benign and malignant tumors	
Features	**Benign**	**Malignant**
Structure	Resemblance to normal cells (well differentiated)	Abnormal; less similarity to normal cells (anaplastic)
Growth rate	Slow	Rapid
Mitoses	Few	Relatively common
Growth	Usually expansive	Invasive
Growth duration	May stop growing	Rarely stop growing
Encapsulation	Usually	Rarely
Metastasis	None	Frequent
Effect on host	Slight harm, due to location or complication	Significant harm, due to invasion and metastasis

Cancer Classification

From a histological standpoint there are hundreds of different cancers, which are grouped into six major categories:

➢ Carcinoma
➢ Sarcoma
➢ Myeloma
➢ Leukaemia
➢ Lymphoma
➢ Mixed types

Carcinoma

Carcinomas are malignancies of epithelial tissue. Epithelial tissue is the tissue that lines the outer surface of the body and lines the internal cavities such as gastrointestinal tract, respiratory tract, genitourinary tract, etc. Such malignancies account for 80 to 90 percent of all cancer cases. Carcinomas are divided into two major subtypes: Adenocarcinoma, which occurs in mucous membranes or glands and squamous cell carcinoma, which originates in the squamous epithelium.

Examples

➢ Adenocarcinoma breast
➢ Squamous cell carcinoma skin
➢ Carcinoma lung.

Sarcoma

Sarcoma refers to cancer that originates in supportive and connective tissues such as bones, tendons, cartilage, muscle, and fat.

Examples of sarcomas are:

➢ Osteogenic sarcoma (bone)
➢ Chondrosarcoma (cartilage)
➢ Leiomyosarcoma (smooth muscle)
➢ Fibrosarcoma (fibrous tissue)
➢ Liposarcoma (adipose tissue)

Leukemia

Leukemias are cancers of the bone marrow:
➤ Myeloid leukemia (granulocyte white blood cells)
➤ Lymphatic leukemia (lymphocytes)
➤ Polycythaemia vera (malignancy of RBC)

Lymphoma

Lymphomas develop in lymph nodes.

Mixed Types

The type components may be within one category or from different categories. Some examples are:
➤ Adenosquamous carcinoma
➤ Mixed mesodermal tumor
➤ Carcinosarcoma
➤ Teratocarcinoma

Causes

The majority of cancers, some 90–95% of cases, are due to genetic mutations resulting from environmental and lifestyle factors. The remaining 5–10% are due to inherited genetic defects.

Cancer is caused by changes (mutations) to the DNA within cells. The DNA inside a cell is packaged into a large number of individual genes, each of which regulates the functioning of the cell as well as regulate its growth and division. Errors in the instructions can cause the cell to stop its normal function and may allow a cell to become cancerous. Normal cells know when to stop growing so that there is just the right number of each type of cell. Cancer cells lose the controls (tumor suppressor genes) that tell them when to stop growing. A mutation in a tumor suppressor gene allows cancer cells to continue growing and accumulating.

What Causes Gene mutations?

Gene mutations can occur for several reasons, for instance:
➤ **Gene mutations at birth.** One may be born with mutation in genes that one inherits from parents. This type of mutation accounts for a small percentage of cancers.
➤ **Gene mutations that occur after birth.** Most gene mutations occur after birth and are not inherited. A number of factors can cause gene mutations, such as smoking, radiation, viruses, cancer-causing chemicals, obesity, hormones, chronic inflammation.

Gene mutations occur frequently during normal cell growth. However, cells contain a mechanism that recognizes when a mistake occurs and repairs the mistake. Occasionally, a mistake is missed. This could cause a cell to become cancerous.

Risk Factors

1. **Age:** Advancing age is the most important risk factor for cancer. According to the most recent statistical data median age of a cancer diagnosis is 66 years. But

the disease can occur at any age. For example, bone cancer is most frequently diagnosed among people under age 20 years. And 10 percent of leukaemias are diagnosed in children and adolescents under 20 years of age. Some types of cancer, such as neuroblastoma, are more common in children or adolescents than in adults.

2. **Tobacco smoke:** Tobacco smoke is responsible for 90% of lung cancer. It also causes cancer in the larynx and esophagus. Tobacco smoke contains over fifty known carcinogens, including nitrosamines and polycyclic aromatic hydrocarbons. Betel nut chewing can cause oral cancer.

3. **Infection:** Worldwide approximately 18% of cancer deaths are related to infectious diseases. This proportion ranges from a high of 25% in Africa to less than 10% in the developed world. Viruses are the usual infectious agents that cause cancer. Bacterial infection may also increase the risk of cancer, as seen in *Helicobacter pylori* induced gastric carcinoma.

4. **Radiation:** Radiation exposure such as ultraviolet radiation and radioactive material is a risk factor for cancer. Many skin cancers are due to ultraviolet radiation, mostly from sunlight.

5. **Physical agents:** Some substances cause cancer primarily through their physical, rather than chemical effects. A prominent example of this is prolonged exposure to inhalation of asbestos by miners which is a known cause of lung cancer.

6. **Hormones:** Hormones are important agents in sex-related cancers, such as cancer of the breast, endometrium, prostate, ovary and testis.

7. **Autoimmune diseases:** There is an association between coeliac disease and cancer. Rates of gastrointestinal cancers are increased in people with Crohn's disease and ulcerative colitis, due to chronic inflammation.

Pathogenesis of Cancer

➤ Regardless of difference in types of cancer histologically, there is a common pathophysiological process of malignant tumors or cancer development.

➤ The commonly accepted basis of the pathogenesis of cancer is the damage to the genetic apparatus of cells.

Cancer is fundamentally a disease of tissue growth dysregulation. In order for a normal cell to transform into a cancer cell, the genes that regulate cell growth and differentiation must be altered.

The cell division is regulated by two broad categories of genes:

1. **Proto-oncogenes** are genes that promote normal cell growth and reproduction. Environmental factors alter a proto-oncogene to oncogene. An oncogene is a gene that has the potential to cause cancer. In tumor cells, these genes are expressed at high levels (Fig. 11.2).

2. **Tumor suppressor** genes are genes that inhibit cell division and survival.

Malignant transformation can occur through the formation of oncogenes, or by disabling of tumor suppressor genes. Typically, changes in multiple genes are required to transform a normal cell into a cancer cell.

During normal cell division, when critical functions are altered and malfunctioning, the cell will undergo a programmed form of rapid cell death (apoptosis). Activated oncogenes can cause those cells designated for apoptosis to survive and proliferate instead.

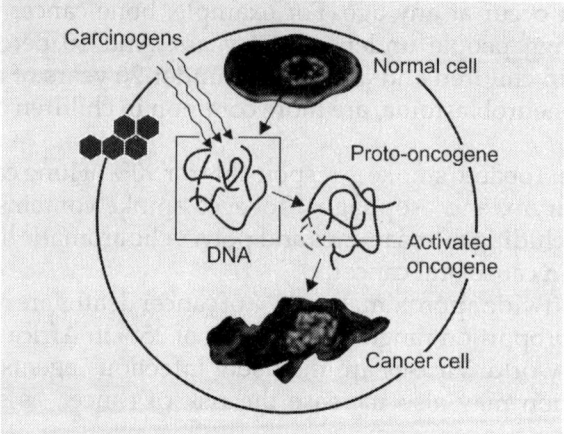

Fig. 11.2: Transformation of proto-oncogene to oncogene initiates development of cancer

STEPS IN INITIATION AND PROGRESSION OF CANCER (FIG. 11.3)

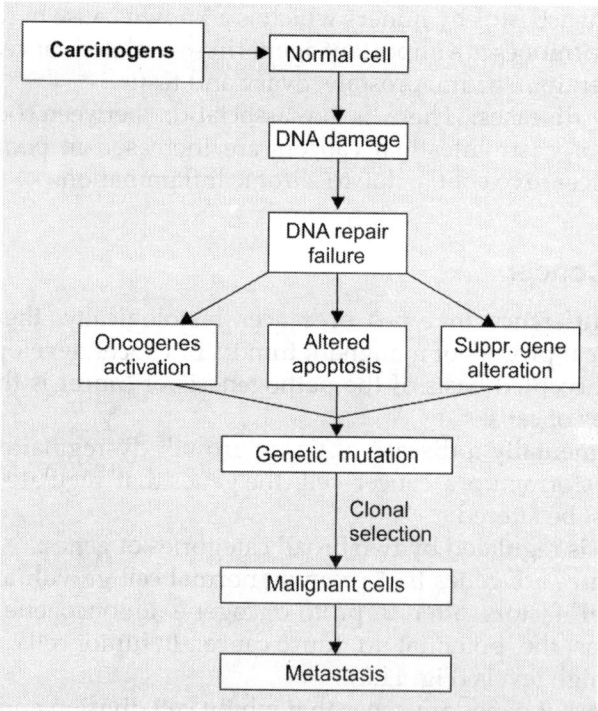

Fig. 11.3: Steps in the development of a normal cell into cancer cells

First Step: Mutation and Tumor Initiation

As a result of formation of an oncogene or inhibition of the suppression, a cell undergoes genetic mutation. Genetic mutation in a single cell results into abnormal proliferation of that cell known as tumor cell.

Second Step: Cell Proliferation

The mutated cells have some selective advantage over normal cell as such cells show rapid growth and division. The descendants of a cell bearing such additional mutation will consequently become dominant within the tumor population.

Third Step: Clonal Selection and Malignancy

➢ Cell proliferation of tumor then leads to new clone of tumor cells with increased growth rate or other properties (such as survival, invasion, or metastasis) that confer a selective advantage. The process is called clonal selection.
➢ Clonal selection continues throughout tumor development, so tumors continuously become more rapid-growing and increasingly malignant.

Fourth Step: Metastasis

➢ **Metastasis** is a complex process in which cancer cells break away from the primary tumor and circulate through the bloodstream or lymphatic system to other sites in the body.
➢ At new sites, the cells continue to multiply and eventually form additional tumors comprised of cells that reflect the tissue of origin.

HALLMARKS OF CANCER CELLS (FIG.11.4)

When a normal cell is transformed into a cancer cell, it develops certain characteristics which help it to undergo unlimited growth and proliferation as well as helps in its metastasis.

1. Self-sufficiency in Growth Signals

Typically, normal cells of the body require hormones and other growth factors that act as signals for them to grow and divide. Cancer cells, however, have the ability to grow without these external signals. There are multiple ways in which cancer cells can do this:
  i. Cancerous cells may themselves produce growth factors.
  ii. Cancer cells may permanently activate growth signalling pathways.
  iii. Cancer cells may destroy the switch off signalling mechanism that stops excessive growth.

2. Insensitivity to Anti-growth Signals

The cell cycle of normal cell division is tightly regulated at various stages. These processes are orchestrated by proteins known as tumor suppressor genes. The cell division will halt division if DNA is damaged. In cancer, these tumor suppressor proteins are altered so that they do not effectively prevent cell division, even when the cell has severe abnormalities.

3. Evading Programmed Cell Death

Normal cells have the ability to 'self-destruct'; a process known as apoptosis. This is required for organisms to grow and develop properly. Apoptosis is initiated when a cell is damaged or infected. Cancer cells, however, lose this ability; even though cells

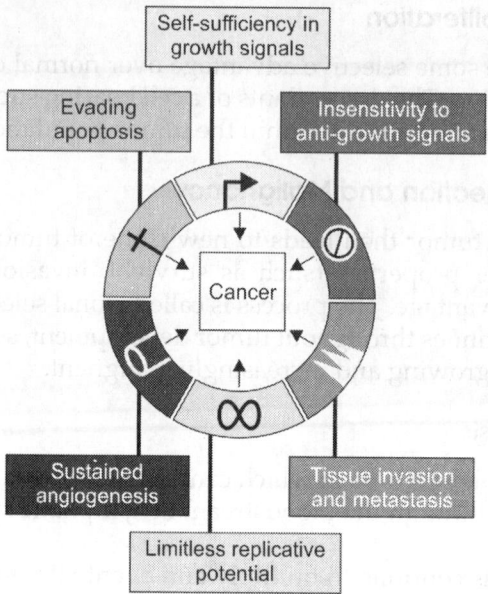

Fig. 11.4: The hallmarks of cancer

may become grossly abnormal, they do not undergo apoptosis. The cancer cells may do this by altering the mechanisms that detect the damage or abnormalities.

4. Limitless Replicative Potential

Normal cells of the body do not have the ability to divide indefinitely. They can have a limited number of divisions before the cells become unable to divide further. Mammalian cells have an intrinsic program, that limits their multiplication to about 60–70 doublings, at which point they reach a stage of senescence. The cause of this barrier is primarily due to the DNA at the end of chromosomes, known as telomeres. Telomeric DNA shortens with every cell division, until it becomes so short it activates senescence, so the cell stops dividing. Cancer cells bypass this barrier by manipulating enzymes (telomerase) to increase the length of telomeres. Thus, they can divide indefinitely, without initiating senescence.

5. Sustained Angiogenesis

Angiogenesis is the process by which new blood vessels are formed. Normal tissues of the body have blood vessels running through them that deliver nutrients and oxygen and remove waste products of tissue metabolism. Normally new blood vessels are formed during wound repair and during the female reproductive cycle. An expanding tumor requires new blood vessels to deliver adequate nutrients and oxygen to the cancer cells (Fig. 11.5). This is achieved by cancer cells' ability to orchestrate production of new vasculature by activating the 'angiogenic switch' and increasing the production of factors that promote blood vessel formation.

6. Tissue Invasion and Metastasis

A key feature that distinguishes cancer cells from all other cells is the capability to spread throughout the body by two related mechanisms: Invasion and metastasis.

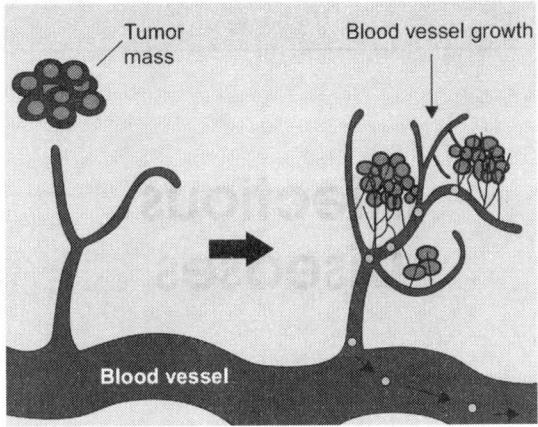

Fig. 11.5: Tumor angiogenesis

INVASION

The capacity for tumor cells to disrupt the basement membrane and penetrate underlying stroma, is the distinguishing feature of malignancy (Fig.11.6).

Invasion refers to the direct extension and penetration by cancer cells into neighbouring tissues. The proliferation of transformed cells and the progressive increase in tumor size eventually leads to a breach in the barriers between tissues, leading to tumor extension into adjacent tissue. Local invasion is also the first stage in the process that leads to the development of secondary tumors or metastases.

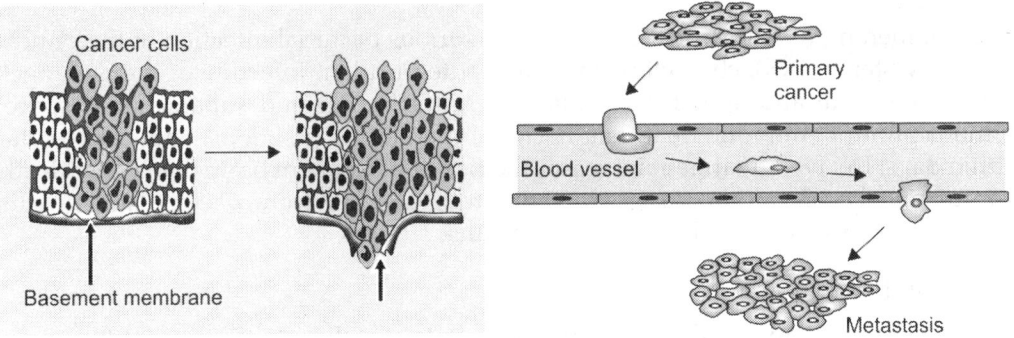

Fig. 11.6: Cancer cells' local invasion (left) and metastasis (right)

METASTASIS

Metastasis, meaning to move to another place, describes the ability of cancer cells to penetrate into lymphatic and blood vessels, circulate through these systems and invade normal tissues elsewhere in the body. The ability of cancer cells to migrate from a primary site of disease is attributed to the mutation of genes that regulate the production of proteins that normally *tether (fasten) cells to their surrounding tissues.* Decreased synthesis by cancer cells of a number of substances that bind them to neighbouring cells, together with the abnormal synthesis of enzymes capable of degrading the bonds between cells and tissues, allow cancer cells to escape the primary tumor site.

Infectious Diseases

Over the previous centuries, global pandemics of infectious diseases, such as smallpox, cholera, and influenza, periodically threatened the survival of entire populations. By the mid-twentieth century, safe, effective, and affordable vaccines and the increasing availability of antibiotics had further reduced the toll of infectious diseases in high income countries. Not until the second half of the twentieth century did large-scale efforts begin to better control infectious diseases in low- and middle-income countries, where the infectious disease burden was greatest and highly varied. A survey in 1998 revealed that infectious diseases accounted for about 50% of disease burden in India. Not much has changed in 2020.

MENINGITIS

Bacterial meningitis is the most common and serious bacterial infection of the central nervous system (CNS), characterized by an acute purulent infection of the meninges around the brain and spinal cord (pia mater, arachnoid) and subarachnoid space. Without prompt antibiotic treatment bacterial meningitis is serious, and can be fatal within days. Delayed treatment increases the risk of permanent brain damage or death Approximately 1.2 million cases are estimated to suffer from bacterial meningitis annually worldwide, resulting in 135,000 deaths.

The Meninges

The meninges comprise three membranes that, together with the cerebrospinal fluid, enclose and protect the brain and spinal cord. The pia mater is a very delicate impermeable membrane that firmly adheres to the surface of the brain. The arachnoid mater is a loosely fitting sac on top of the pia mater. The subarachnoid space separates the arachnoid and pia mater membranes and is filled with cerebrospinal fluid. The outermost membrane, the dura mater, is a thick durable membrane, which is attached to both the arachnoid membrane and the skull (Fig. 12.1).

Symptoms and Signs

Early meningitis symptoms may mimic upper respiratory tract infection. Symptoms may develop over several hours or over a few days. Possible signs and symptoms in anyone older than the age of 2 include:

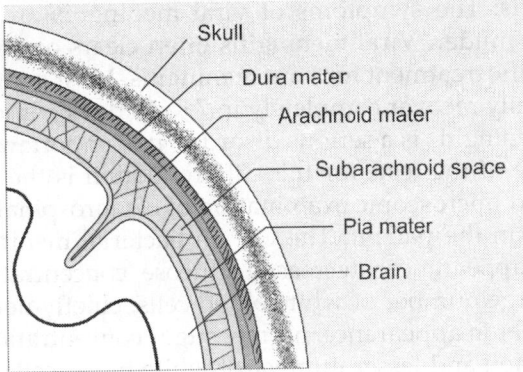

Fig. 12.1: The meninges

➤ Sudden high fever
➤ Stiff neck
➤ Severe headache
➤ Headache with nausea or vomiting
➤ Confusion or difficulty concentrating
➤ Seizures
➤ Sleepiness or difficulty waking
➤ Photophobia (sensitivity to light)
➤ No appetite or thirst
➤ Skin rash (sometimes, such as in meningococcal meningitis).

Causes

i. **Bacterial meningitis:** Bacteria that enter the bloodstream and travel to the brain and spinal cord cause acute bacterial meningitis. Pneumococcus or meningococcus type of bacteria are causative organisms (Fig. 12.2).

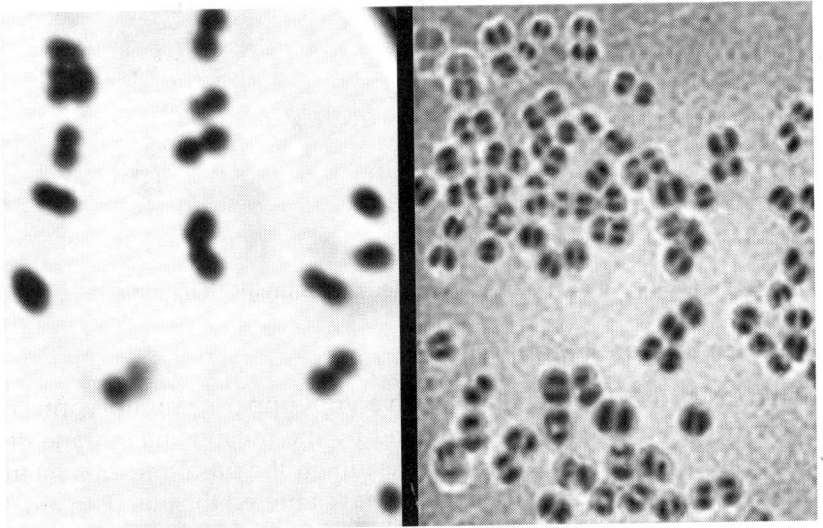

Fig. 12.2: Pneumococci (left) and meningococci (right)

ii. **Viral meningitis:** The symptoms of viral meningitis are same as in bacterial meningitis, but milder. Viral meningitis often clears on its own. In most cases, there is no specific treatment for viral meningitis. Most people who get mild viral meningitis usually recover completely in 7 to 10 days without treatment.

Since, bacterial meningitis is a serious disorder, it is important to differentiate from viral meningitis. One of the tests for this differentiation is the physical appearance, chemical analysis and microscopic examination of cerebrospinal fluid (CSF) obtained by lumbar puncture in the patient. The CSF in bacterial meningitis is characterised by being turbid in appearance, decreased glucose concentration, increase protein concentration and large number of white blood cells, chiefly neutrophils. The CSF in viral meningitis is clear in appearance, normal sugar concentration, only mild increase in protein concentration and lesser number of white blood cells, chiefly lymphocytes (Table 12.1 and Fig. 12.3)

Table 12.1	Physical appearance and chemical composition of CSF in bacterial and viral meningitis			
	Appearance	*WBC (per cmm)*	*Protein (mg/dL)*	*Glucose (mg/dL)*
Normal	Clear	<8	15–45	50–80
Bacterial meningitis	Turbid	>1000–2000	>200	<40
Viral meningtis	Clear	<300 Lymphocytic predominance	<200	Normal

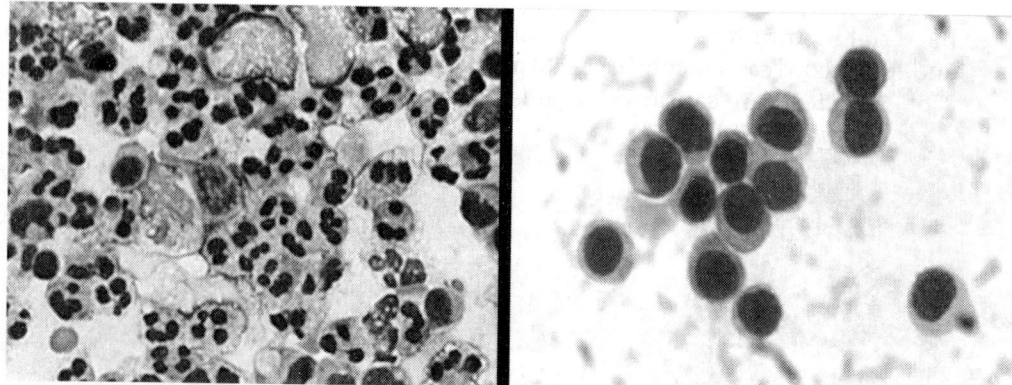

Fig. 12.3: Microscopic appearance of CSF in bacterial meningitis (left) and viral meningitis (right)

Pathogenesis of Bacterial Meningitis

In most of the cases, the disorder starts with a viral upper respiratory infection which breaks down the protective barrier provided by the mucous membrane of the nasal cavity. As a result, bacteria that normally reside on the nasal mucous membrane are able to enter the blood stream. Once bacteria have entered the bloodstream, they enter the subarachnoid space in places where the blood–brain barrier is relatively weak, i.e. the choroid plexus.

The cerebrospinal fluid present in the subarachnoid space is an ideal medium for proliferation of bacteria because it has enough nutrients and very few phagocytic cells. Cells of the innate immune system of CNS (microglia and astrocytes) located in the choroid plexus and ependyma, detect bacteria and secrete cytokines and chemokines which attract circulating granulocytes into CSF. Granulocytes and macrophages contain powerful lysosomal enzymes used to kill the bacteria, but these cells have short lifespan. On senescence, these cells release proteolytic enzymes into cerebral interstitial space and damage the brain tissue and blood vessels (vasculitis). So the brain damage in bacterial meningitis is partly due to bacteria and partly by inflammatory response. The most dangerous complication of bacterial meningitis is increased intracranial pressure from cerebral edema. Cerebral edema results from greater permeability of blood–brain barrier, increased cerebral hypoxia and cellular toxicity. Increased intracranial pressure, in turn, causes decreased cerebral perfusion, ischemia, hypoxia and neuronal necrosis (Fig. 12.4).

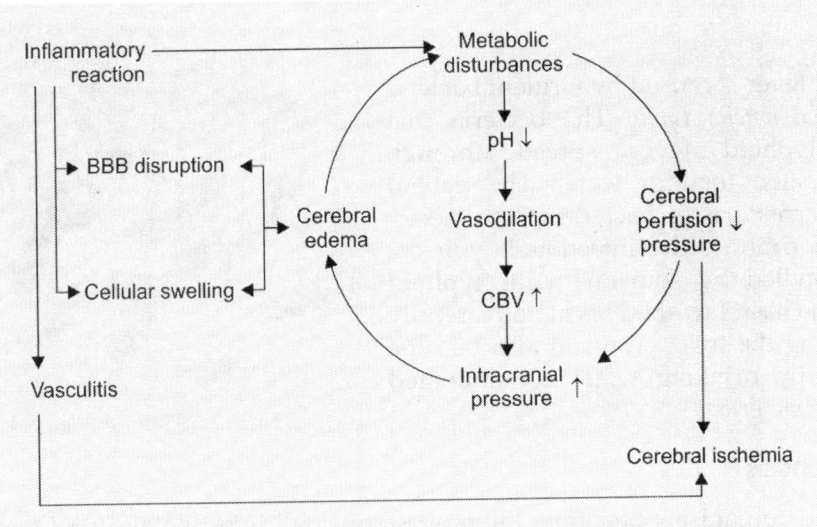

Fig. 12.4: Mechanisms of increased intracranial pressure and cerebral ischemia in bacterial meningitis (BBB, blood–brain barrier; CBV, cerebral blood volume)

Complications

Meningitis complications can be severe. The longer the delay in start of treatment, greater is the brain damage and other complications, including:

➢ Hearing loss.
➢ Cortical blindness.
➢ Other cranial nerve dysfunction.
➢ Paralysis.
➢ Muscular hypertonia.
➢ Ataxia.
➢ Mental retardation.
➢ Kidney failure
➢ Death.

▎TYPHOID FEVER

Typhoid, also called typhoid fever, occurs all over the world. In 2015, 12.5 million new cases worldwide were reported. The risk of death may be as high as 20% without treatment. In 2015, it resulted in about 149,000 deaths worldwide. The disease is endemic in India, Southeast Asia, Africa and South America.

Symptoms and Signs

> In the first week, the body temperature rises slowly, and fever fluctuations are seen with malaise, headache, and cough.
> In the second week, high fever around 40°C (104°F). The abdomen is distended and painful in the right lower quadrant. The spleen and liver are enlarged (hepatosplenomegaly).
> In the third week of typhoid fever, a number of **complications** can occur:
> + *Intestinal haemorrhage* due to bleeding in congested Peyer's patches;
> + *Intestinal perforation* in the distal ileum, a very serious complication and is frequently fatal.
> + *Septicaemia* or *peritonitis*.

Cause

Typhoid fever is caused by virulent bacteria called *Salmonella typhi*. The bacteria that cause typhoid fever spread through contaminated food or water. The patient or the carrier passes bacteria in the faeces. You can contract the infection if you eat food handled by someone with typhoid fever who hasn't washed his hands carefully after using the toilet. You can also become infected by drinking water contaminated with the bacteria.

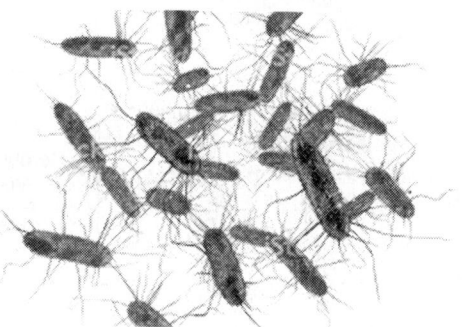

Fig. 12.5: *Salmonella typhi*

Pathogenesis

Salmonella organisms penetrate the mucosa of small intestine and proliferate in the mucosal epithelial cells. Next, the bacteria proliferate in the Payer's patches (sub-mucosal collection of lymphoid tissue) (Fig. 12.6) of the lower small intestine from where systemic dissemination occurs to the reticuloendothelial system of liver and spleen.

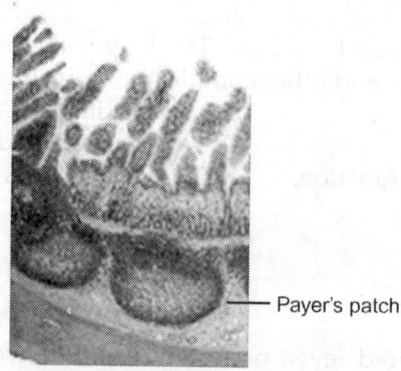

Payer's patch

Fig. 12.6: Payer's patch in ileum

For a period varying from 1 to 3 weeks, the organism multiplies within these organs. Invasion of the mucosa causes the epithelial cells to synthesise and release various proinflammatory cytokines responsible for the most of the symptoms of typhoid fever. Ulceration over Payer's patches account for complications such as bleeding, perforation and peritonitis (Fig. 12.7). Proliferation in reticuloendothelial system leads to enlargement and congestion of the spleen and liver. Figure 12.8 illustrates the pathophysiology of typhoid fever.

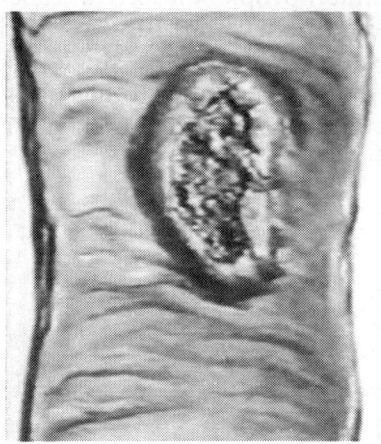

Fig. 12.7: Typhoid ulcer in small intestine

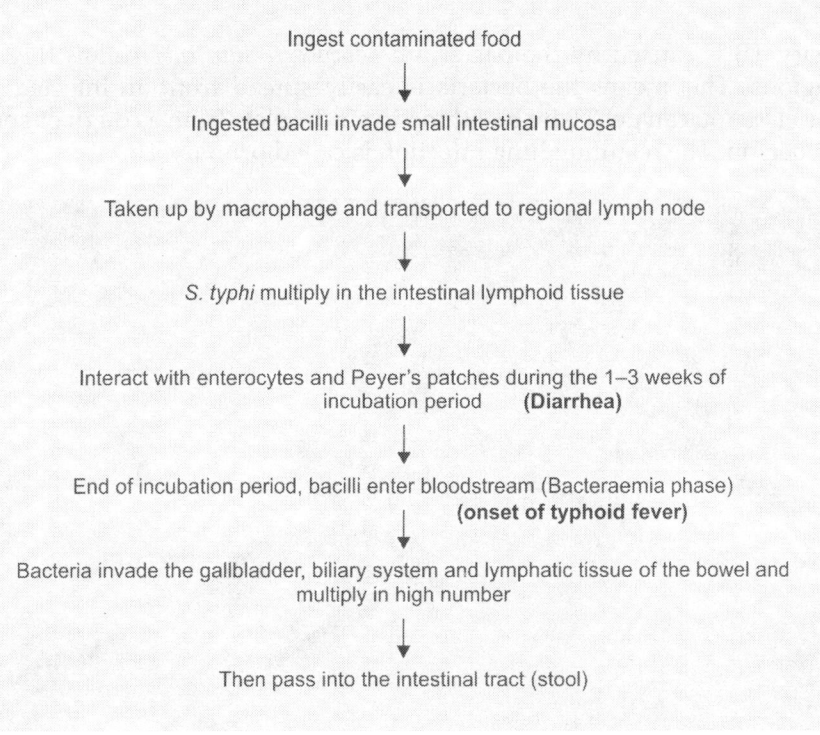

Fig. 12.8: Pathophysiology of typhoid fever

Complications

- ➤ Intestinal hemorrhage
- ➤ Intestinal perforation
- ➤ Septicaemia
- ➤ Peritonitis
- ➤ Death

┃TUBERCULOSIS

In 2018, an estimated 10 million people fell ill with tuberculosis (TB) worldwide. A total of 1.5 million people died from TB in 2018. Worldwide, TB is one of the top 10 causes of death and the leading cause from a single infectious agent. Tuberculosis generally affects the lungs, but can also affect other parts of the body. About 25% of TB patients of the world are Indians. In India, each year, approx. 220,000 deaths are reported due to tuberculosis.

Pulmonary Tuberculosis

Symptoms and Signs

- ➤ Cough up sputum
- ➤ Cough up blood
- ➤ Consistent low-grade fever
- ➤ Night sweats
- ➤ Chest pains
- ➤ Unexplained weight loss

Cause

Pulmonary TB is caused by the bacterium *Mycobacterium tuberculosis* (Fig. 12.9). TB is contagious. This means the bacteria is easily spread from an infected person to someone else. You can get TB by breathing in air droplets from a cough or sneeze of an infected person. The resulting lung infection is called primary TB.

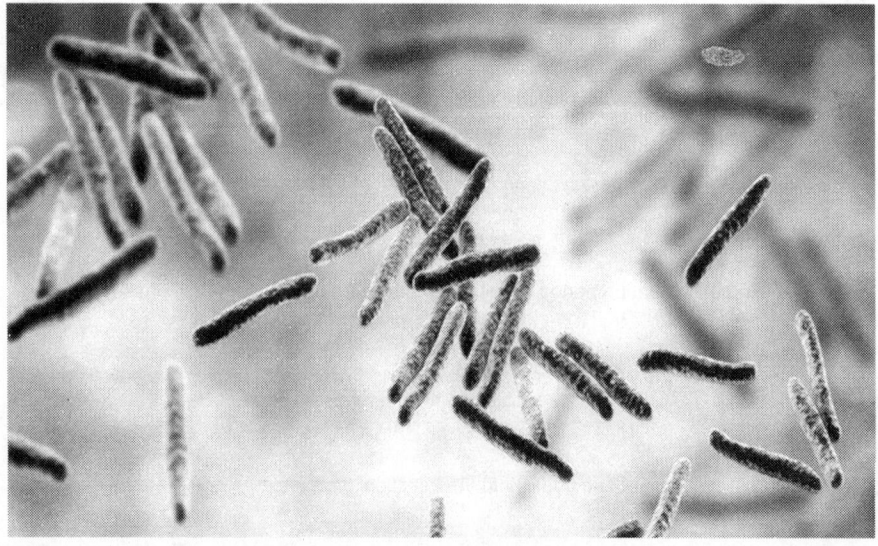

Fig. 12.9: *Mycobacterium tuberculosis*

Pathogenesis

The characteristic pathologic changes depend on the type of infection:
- **Primary pulmonary TB** (primary exposure) is characterized by the Ghon complex which consists of
  1. Subpleural focus of tubercular inflammation.
  2. Infected (inflamed) lymph nodes draining the primary subpleural lesion.
- **Secondary pulmonary TB** (reactivation) is characterized by a focus of infection and granuloma formation usually in the apex of the lung. The small granulomas (tubercles) eventually coalesce to form larger areas of consolidation with central caseating necrosis. Regional lymph nodes contain caseating granulomas.
- **Progressive pulmonary TB**: Primary or secondary TB may go on to heal as caseating granulomas are replaced by fibrosis and calcification. However, if the case does not heal spontaneously or with therapy, the disease progress to form cavities or spread to other parts of the lung and other organs of the body through lymphatic channels and the blood stream.

Primary Tuberculosis

The tubercle bacilli establish infection in the lungs after they are carried in droplets small enough (5 to 10 microns) to reach the alveolar spaces. If the defense system of the host fails to eliminate the infection, the bacilli proliferate inside alveolar macrophages and eventually kill the cells. The infected macrophages produce cytokines and chemokines that attract other phagocytic cells, including monocytes, other alveolar macrophages and neutrophils, which eventually form a nodular granulomatous structure called the tubercle (*see* Chapter 2). If the bacterial replication is not controlled, the tubercle enlarges and the bacilli enter local draining lymph nodes. This leads to lymphadenopathy, a characteristic clinical manifestation of primary tuberculosis. The lesion produced by the expansion of the tubercle into the lung parenchyma and lymph node involvement is called the Ghon complex (Fig. 12.10).

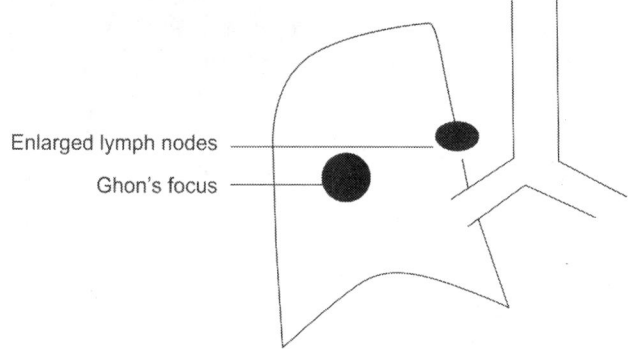

Enlarged lymph nodes

Ghon's focus

Fig. 12.10: The Ghon's complex

Unchecked bacterial growth may lead to haematogenous spread of bacilli to produce disseminated TB in various vital organs of the body. Disseminated disease with lesions resembling millet seeds is termed miliary TB (Fig. 12.11). In the absence of treatment, death ensues in 80% of cases. The remaining patients develop chronic disease or recover. Chronic disease is characterized by repeated episodes of healing by fibrotic changes around the lesions and tissue breakdown. Complete spontaneous eradication of the bacilli is rare.

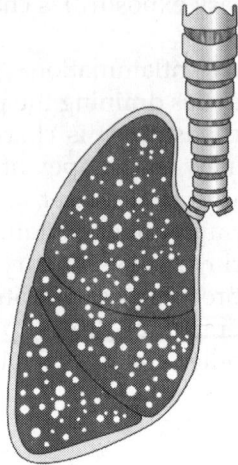

Fig. 12.11: Miliary tuberculosis lungs

Reactivation Disease

Reactivation TB results from proliferation of a previously dormant bacterium seeded at the time of the primary infection. Among individuals with latent infection and no underlying medical problems, reactivation disease occurs in 5 to 10 per cent. It is not clear what specific host factors maintain the infection in a latent state and what triggers the latent infection to become overt. The disease process in reactivation TB tends to be localized (in contrast to primary disease): There is little regional lymph node involvement and less caseation. The lesion typically occurs at the lung apices, and disseminated disease is unusual unless the host is severely immunosuppressed. It is generally believed that successfully contained latent TB confers protection against subsequent TB exposure. In many people, the infection waxes and wanes. Tissue destruction and necrosis are often balanced by healing and fibrosis. Affected tissue is replaced by scarring and cavities filled with caseous necrotic material. Tissue destruction and necrosis are often balanced by healing and fibrosis. Affected tissue is replaced by scarring and cavities filled with caseous necrotic material (Fig. 12.12). During active disease, some of these cavities are joined to the bronchi and this material can be coughed up. The sputum contains living bacteria, and thus can spread the infection (Fig. 12.13).

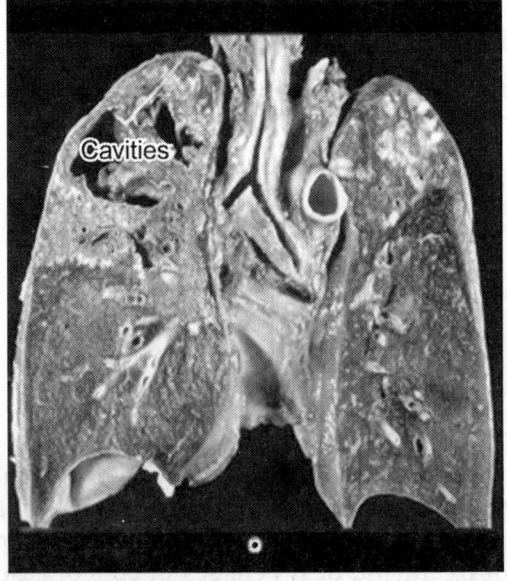

Fig. 12.12: Tuberculosis lungs showing cavities

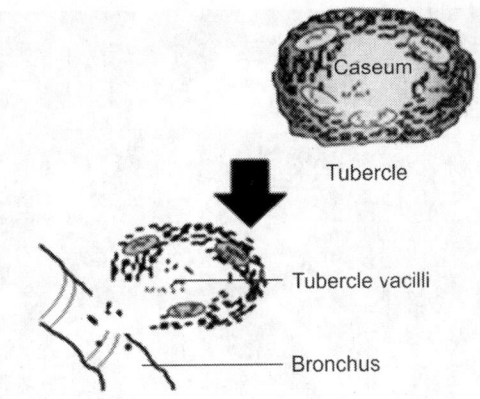

Fig. 12.13: Tubercular cavity opening into a bronchus

Risk factors

➤ Contact with a patient of TB
➤ Live in crowded or unclean living conditions
➤ Have poor nutrition

Complications

➤ Hemoptysis
➤ Pleurisy
➤ Pleural effusion
➤ Empyema
➤ Pneumothorax

➤ Bronchiectasis
➤ Laryngitis
➤ Cor pulmonale (congestive heart failure)

▌LEPROSY

Leprosy currently affects approximately a quarter of a million people throughout the world, with the majority of these cases being reported from India. India is currently running one of the largest leprosy eradication programs in the world. Despite this, 120,000 to 130,000 new cases of leprosy are reported every year in India. This is 58.8% of the global total of new cases. Leprosy colonies exist throughout India. These are typically made up of patients that have moved to the colony often from a significant distance away, along with their children and grandchildren. Leprosy is a curable disease.

Leprosy, also known as Hansen's disease, is a chronic infectious disease caused by *Mycobacterium leprae* (Fig. 12.14). The disease mainly affects the skin, the peripheral nerves, mucosal surfaces of the upper respiratory tract and the eyes. Leprosy is known to occur at all ages ranging from early infancy to very old age. Leprosy is curable and early treatment averts most disabilities.

Transmission

The exact mechanism of transmission of leprosy is not known. At least until recently, the most widely held belief was that the disease was transmitted by contact between cases of leprosy and healthy persons. More recently the possibility of transmission by the respiratory route is gaining ground.

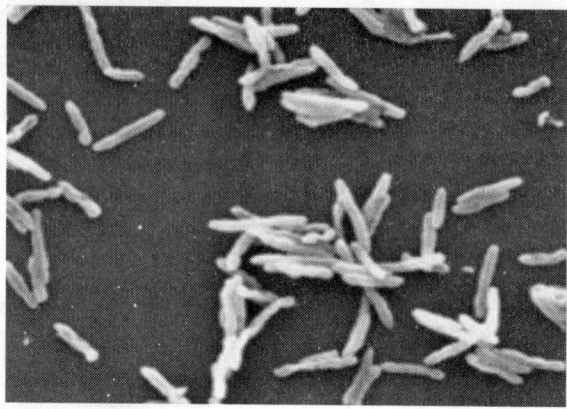

Fig. 12.14: *Mycobacterium leprae*

Symptoms and Signs

The skin lesion is a characteristic feature of leprosy (Fig. 12.15). The skin lesion can be single or multiple, usually less pigmented than the surrounding normal skin. Sometimes the lesion is reddish or copper-coloured. A variety of skin lesions may be seen but macules (flat), papules (raised), or nodules are common. Sensory loss is a typical feature of leprosy. The skin lesion may show loss of sensation to pin pick and/ or light touch. Thickened nerves, mainly peripheral nerve trunks, constitute another feature of leprosy. A thickened nerve is often accompanied by other signs as a result of damage to the nerve. These may be loss of sensation in the skin and weakness of muscles supplied by the affected nerve.

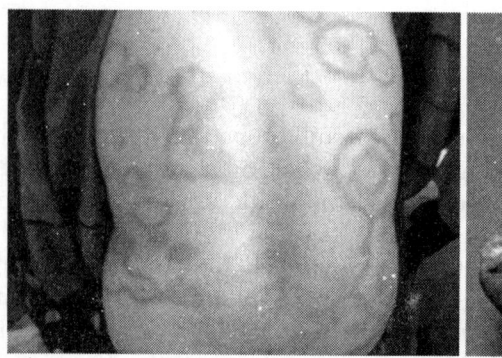
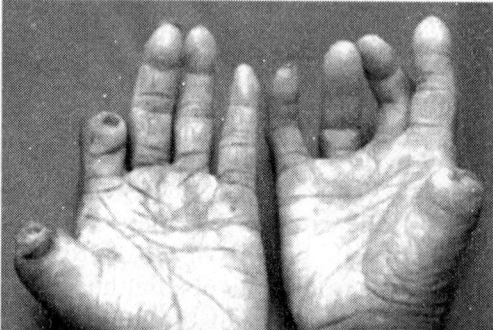

Tuberculoid type   Lapromatous type

Fig. 12.15: The two types of leprosy

Pathogenesis

Leprosy bacilli multiply in macrophages in the skin and Schwann cells of the nerves. Two forms of leprosy are known:

One form is "tuberculoid type which is a mild form. *M. leprae* multiplies at the site of entry, usually the skin, invading and colonizing Schwann cells. The microbe then induces T-helper lymphocytes, epithelioid cells, and giant cell infiltration of the skin, causing infected individuals to exhibit large flattened patches with raised and elevated red edges on their skin (Fig. 12.15). These patches have dry, pale, hairless centers, accompanied by a loss of sensation on the skin. The loss of sensation may develop as a result of invasion of the peripheral sensory nerves.

The second form of leprosy, the "lepromatous type", causes serious disfigurement is more virulent. In this form, the microbes proliferate within the macrophages as well as within the epithelial tissues of the face and ear lobes. Extensive penetration of this microbe may lead to severe body damage; for example, the loss of bones, fingers, and toes, nose (Fig. 12.15).

Risk Factor

Prolonged contact with a patient of leprosy.

Complications

➢ The most severe complications result from the peripheral neuropathy, which causes deterioration of the sense of touch and a corresponding inability to feel pain and temperature.
➢ Patients may unknowingly burn, cut, or otherwise harm themselves. Repeated damage may lead to loss of digits.
➢ Muscle weakness can result in deformities (e.g. clawing of the 4th and 5th fingers caused by ulnar nerve involvement, foot drop caused by peroneal nerve involvement).
➢ Papules and nodules can be particularly disfiguring on the face.
➢ *Feet:* Plantar ulcers with secondary infection are a major cause of morbidity, making walking painful.
➢ *Nose:* Damage to the nasal mucosa can result in chronic nasal congestion and nosebleeds and, if untreated, erosion and collapse of the nasal septum.
➢ *Eyes:* Iritis may lead to glaucoma, and corneal insensitivity may lead to scarring and blindness.
➢ *Sexual function:* Men with lepromatous leprosy may have erectile dysfunction and infertility. The infection can reduce testosterone and sperm production by the testes.
➢ *Kidneys:* Amyloidosis and consequent renal failure occasionally occur in lepromatous leprosy.

URINARY TRACT INFECTION

Urinary tract infections (UTIs) are some of the most common bacterial infections, affecting 150 million people each year worldwide. About 40% of women and 12% of men experience at least one symptomatic UTI during their lifetime, and as many as 40% of affected women show recurrent UTI. A urinary tract infection (UTI) is an infection in any part of urinary system—kidneys, ureters, bladder and urethra. Most infections involve the lower urinary tract—the bladder and the urethra. Women are at greater risk of developing a UTI than are men, since they have very short urethra. Urinary tract infections (UTIs) are the most common outpatient infections, with a lifetime incidence of 50–60% in adult women. Serious consequences can occur if a UTI spreads to the kidneys.

Symptoms and Signs

Each type of UTI may result in more-specific signs and symptoms, depending on which part of your urinary tract is infected.

Part of urinary tract affected	Signs and symptoms
Kidneys (acute pyelonephritis)	Upper back and side (flank) pain
	High fever
	Shaking and chills
	Nausea
	Vomiting
Bladder (cystitis)	Pelvic pressure
	Lower abdomen discomfort
	Frequent, painful urination
	Blood in urine
Urethra (urethritis)	Burning with urination
	Discharge

Microscopic examination of urine reveals a large number of white blood cells (Fig. 12.16). Microbiological culture helps to identify the causative organism as well as their sensitivity to drugs.

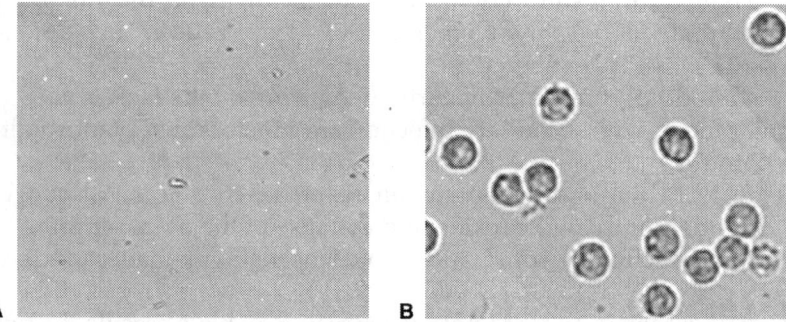

Fig. 12.16: Microscopic examination of urine. (A) Normal; (B). A patient of UTI

Causes

Urinary tract infections typically occur when bacteria enter the urinary tract through the urethra and begin to multiply in the bladder. Although the urinary system is designed to keep out such microscopic invaders, these defences sometimes fail. When that happens, bacteria may take hold and grow into a full-blown infection in the urinary tract. The most common UTIs occur mainly in women and affect the bladder and urethra. *Escherichia coli* (*E. coli*) (Fig. 12.17) from the gut is the cause of 80–85% of community-acquired urinary tract infections.[23]

Risk Factors

Risk factors specific to women for UTIs include:
➤ **Female anatomy.** A woman has a shorter urethra than a man does, which shortens the distance that bacteria must travel to reach the bladder.
➤ **Sexual activity.**
➤ **Menopause.** After menopause, a decline in circulating estrogen causes changes in the urinary tract that make women more vulnerable to infection.
➤ *Urinary tract abnormalities.*

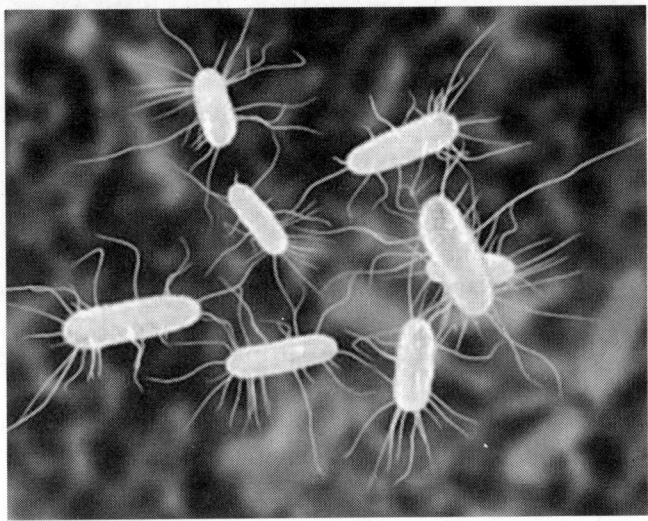

Fig. 12.17: *E. coli*

> *Blockages in the urinary tract.* Urinary obstruction by kidney stones or an enlarged prostate in males increase risk of UTIs.
> Diabetes

Complications

When treated promptly and properly, lower urinary tract infections rarely lead to complications. But left untreated, a urinary tract infection can have serious consequences.
> Recurrent infections, especially in women.
> Permanent kidney damage from an acute or chronic kidney infection (pyelonephritis) due to an untreated UTI.
> Sepsis, a potentially life-threatening complication of an infection, especially if the infection spreads to the kidneys.

GONORRHEA

Gonorrhea, is a sexually transmitted infection (STI). It is a global problem. The World Health Organization estimates that 62 million people are infected annually worldwide. In the United States, it is the second most commonly reported communicable disease and the second most prevalent sexually transmitted infection. In India, its exact prevalence is not known because of non-reporting by the patients.

Symptoms and Signs

In many cases, gonorrhoea infection causes no symptoms. Symptoms, however, can affect many sites in the body, but commonly appear in the genital tract.

Signs and symptoms of gonorrhoea infection in men include:
> Painful urination
> Pus-like discharge from the tip of the penis
> Pain or swelling in one testicle

Signs and symptoms of gonorrhea infection in women include:
➤ Increased vaginal discharge
➤ Painful urination
➤ Vaginal bleeding between periods, such as after vaginal intercourse
➤ Abdominal or pelvic pain

Gonorrhea can also affect these parts of the body:
➤ **Rectum:** Signs and symptoms include anal itching, pus-like discharge from the rectum.
➤ **Eyes:** Gonorrhea that affects the eyes can cause eye pain and pus-like discharge from the eye.
➤ **Throat.** Signs and symptoms of a throat infection might include a sore throat and swollen lymph nodes in the neck.
➤ **Joints.** If one or more joints become infected by bacteria (septic arthritis), the affected joints might be warm, red, swollen and extremely painful, especially during movement.

Cause

Gonorrhoea, is caused by the bacterium *Neisseria gonorrhoeae* (Fig. 12.18).

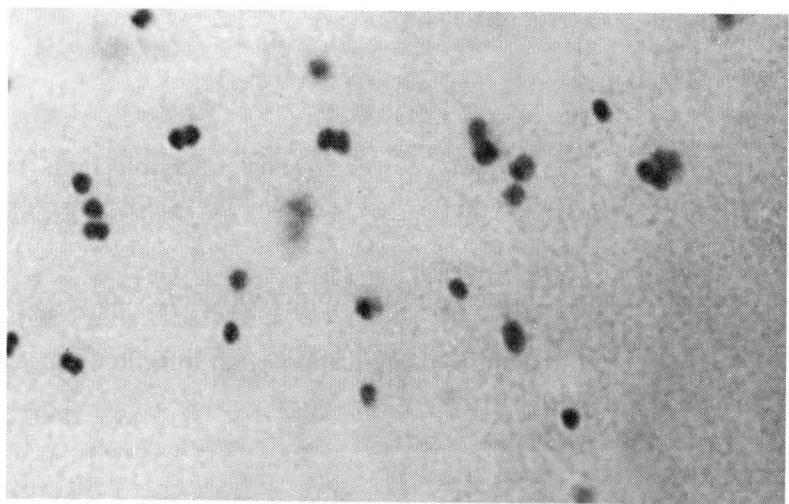

Fig. 12.18: *Neisseria gonorrhoeae*

Pathogenesis

Transmission of infection from one person to another normally occurs during the periods of close physical contact which allow the organisms to pass from the site of infection in one host, to a susceptible mucosal surface in a new one. The infection is usually transmitted during intimate sexual contact, the most common site of infection being the mucosa of the genital tract. In addition, babies born to mothers harbouring gonococci in their genital tract may become infected during passage down the birth canal and may develop gonococcal conjunctivitis.

Neisseria gonorrhoeae is an obligate human pathogen that causes mucosal surface infections of male and female reproductive tracts, pharynx, rectum, and conjunctiva.

Asymptomatic infections in the lower reproductive tract of women can lead to serious, long-term consequences if these infections ascend into the fallopian tube. The damage caused by gonococcal infection and the subsequent inflammatory response produce the condition known as pelvic inflammatory disease (PID). Infection can lead to tubal scarring, occlusion of the oviduct, and loss of critical ciliated cells. These defects interfere with the normal transport of ovum from ovary to the uterus. Consequently, there is increased risk of ectopic pregnancy and infertility.

Complications

Untreated gonorrhea can lead to major complications, such as:
➤ Infertility in women.
➤ Infertility in men.
➤ Infection that spreads to the joints and other areas of your body.
➤ Increased risk of HIV/AIDS.
➤ Complications in babies. Babies who contract gonorrhea from their mothers during birth can develop blindness.

SYPHILIS

Syphilis is a bacterial infection usually spread by sexual contact. The disease starts as a painless sore—typically on your genitals. Syphilis is caused by a bacterium called *Treponema pallidum* (Fig. 12.19). Syphilis spreads from person to person via skin or mucous membrane. During the last 50 years, the prevalence of this disease seems to have decreased.

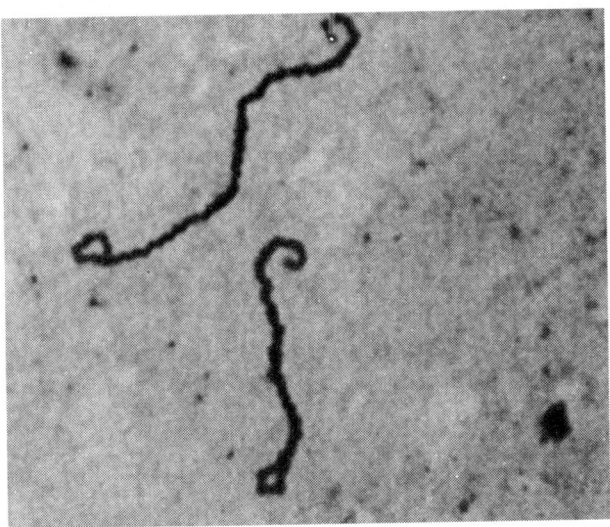

Fig. 12.19: *Treponema pallidum*

After the initial infection, the syphilis bacteria can remain inactive (dormant) in the body for decades before becoming active again. Early syphilis can be cured, sometimes with a single shot of penicillin. Without treatment, syphilis can severely damage the heart, brain or other organs, and can be life-threatening. Syphilis can also be passed from mothers to unborn children.

Symptoms and Signs

Primary syphilis

The first sign of syphilis is a small sore, called a chancre. The sore appears at the spot where the bacteria entered the body. The chancre usually develops about three weeks after exposure. Many people who have syphilis do not notice the chancre because it is usually painless. The chancre will heal on its own within three to six weeks.

Secondary syphilis

Within a few weeks of the original chancre healing, the patient experience a rash that begins on the trunk but eventually covers the entire body. Some people also experience fever, a sore throat and swollen lymph nodes. These signs and symptoms may disappear within a few weeks.

Latent syphilis

In this stage there are no symptoms and it lasts for many years.

Tertiary syphilis

About 15% to 30% of people infected with syphilis who do not get treatment will develop complications known as late (tertiary) syphilis

Tertiary syphilis is the most serious stage of infection and is characterized by three major complications:

➢ **Gummatous syphilis** causes the formation of soft, tumor-like lesions called gummas. These non-cancerous lesions can cause large ulcerative sores on the skin and mouth, and erode tissues of heart, liver, muscles, bones, and other vital organs. Symptoms typically develop between three and 10 years after being infected.

➢ **Cardiovascular syphilis** can cause severe inflammation of the aorta and the development of an aortic aneurysm (the swelling and weakening of the aortic wall). It generally occurs 10 to 30 years after the initial infection.

➢ **Neurosyphilis** affects the central nervous system and usually develops within four to 25 years of an infection. There may be severe neurological disorders including meningitis, degeneration of spinal cord (tabes dorsalis), seizures, personality changes, hallucinations, dementia, schizophrenia, and stroke.

While the syphilis infection can be treated during the tertiary stage, any damage caused to the heart, kidneys, and other organs may be permanent and lead to end-stage organ failure.

HIV/AIDS

Acquired immunodeficiency syndrome (AIDS) is a chronic potentially life-threatening condition caused by human immunodeficiency virus (HIV). The World Health Organization (WHO) estimates that in 2017, about 37 million people, including 1.8 million children (< 15 years), were living with HIV worldwide; of the total, about 25.7 million live in sub-Saharan Africa. More than two million Indians are suffering from HIV/AIDS. By damaging one's immune system, it interferes with the body's ability to various organs that cause disease.

Symptoms and Signs

Symptoms and signs vary with the stage of the disease:

1. **Primary infection (acute HIV)**
   - Fever
   - Headache
   - Muscle aches
   - Joint pains
   - Rash
   - Swollen lymph nodes in the neck
2. **Clinically latent infection (chronic HIV):** There are no symptoms or signs in this stage. This stage may last 10 years.
3. **Symptomatic HIV infection**
   - Fever
   - Fatigue
   - Swollen lymph nodes
   - Weight loss
   - Diarrhoea

Progression to AIDS

This stage occurs when the patient's immune system has been severely damaged. Pathogens that normally cannot attack the human body are now able to enter the body and produce disease. Such bacteria, viruses and fungi are called opportunistic pathogens. Body loses ability to detect and destroy malignant cells. Therefore, the patient is more prone to develop cancer. At this stage, symptoms and signs may include:

- Night sweats
- Recurring fever
- Chronic diarrhea
- Persistent fatigue
- Weight loss

Pathogenesis

The human immunodeficiency virus (HIV) mainly infects the CD4 cells (helper T-cells) in the immune system. Over years of HIV infection, CD4 cell numbers usually drop gradually, but constantly, and the immune system is weakened. When the CD4 cell number falls below 200 mm^3, symptoms of AIDS develop (Fig. 12.20). At this stage complications listed below begin to appear. Due to opportunistic infections/tumor, severe muscle wasting can be observed in the patient.

Spread

HIV infection is transmitted by sexual intercourse. One can also get HIV infection by coming in contact with infected blood directly or through transfusion of infected blood or use of contaminated syringes.

Complications of AIDS

1. **Viral infections,** such as Cytomegalovirus (CMV), herpes simplex, molluscum, contagiosum, herpes zoster, human papillomavirus (HPV), etc
2. **Bacterial infections,** such as recurrent bacterial pneumonia, *Mycobacterium tuberculosis*, Pseudomonas, septicaemia and vasculitis, etc.

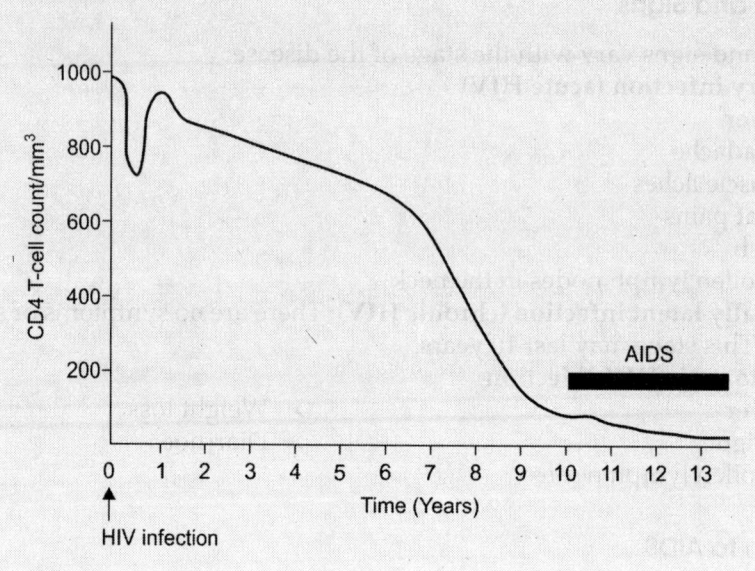

Fig. 12.20: Time course of HIV infection leading to AIDS

3. **Fungal infections,** such as Candida, *Pneumocystis jirovecii,* pneumonia, *Cryptococcus neoformans*
4. **Protozoal infections**
5. **Tumors,** such as Kaposi's sarcoma, primary cerebral lymphoma, high-grade non-Hodgkin lymphoma, carcinoma of the cervix, etc.

Risk Factors

➢ Unprotected sex with a person with HIV/AIDS
➢ Infected blood transfusion
➢ Sharing injection needles with a person with HIV/AIDS

Index